SCHOOL NURSING IN TRANSITION

School nursing in transition

DORIS S. BRYAN, R.N., M.P.H., Ph.D.

*Project Director, School Health and Nutrition Service for the
Oakland Public Schools, U. S. Department of Health, Education,
and Welfare; formerly Consultant in Health and Supervisor
of Nursing Services, Oakland Public Schools, Oakland, California*

With 57 illustrations

THE C. V. MOSBY COMPANY

Saint Louis   1973

Library of Congress Cataloging in Publication Data

Bryan, Doris S   1913-
    School nursing in transition.

        1. School nurses. I. Title. [DNLM: 1. School
nursing. WY113 B915s 1973]
LB3407.B79   371.7′12   73-11115
ISBN 0-8016-0840-6

PREFACE

School Nursing in Transition outlines the principles of interrelation between the nurse in school and children, parents, community, and school workers in this ever-changing world.

Children and youth from preschool through college learn easier, are happier, and can contribute more to society when they are physically, emotionally, mentally, and socially healthy. The potential for optimal physical health for children and youth has never been greater nor the future brighter. Medical science has partially isolated and continues to research the components of physical illness, mental retardation, and emotional disturbance. Children survive infancy in greater numbers, mature earlier, and attain greater stature than did their parents and grandparents.

The demand for school nursing services—from the paraprofessional to the school nurse practitioner—is growing. Nurses are performing different tasks in a variety of settings with a multiplicity of experiences, skills, and educational backgrounds. The social forces affecting school nursing practice continually increase. A glance at any local newspaper or periodical indicates that civil strife, new methods in medicine and education, rebellious youth, increased problems in drug abuse and venereal disease, new legislation, and health manpower shortages are continually affecting pupils, parents, and school and community health personnel. Schools still offer the greatest resource and potential for change.

This book presents an overview of school nursing philosophy, current practices, and patterns of administration. Special emphasis is placed upon redirection of services—learning new methods and techniques based upon a firm foundation of nursing knowledge and skills. It is hoped the nursing student, the practitioner, and the school administrator will all find this book helpful in developing understanding and respect for the school nurse as a professional and as a human being.

The sections on administration of programs, guidelines for implementing new services, and nursing responsibilities and procedures will be helpful and adaptable in a variety of school nursing situations. It is recognized that programs and circumstances differ with the health needs of children, available money, community resources, and educational philosophy.

The hard work, aspirations, dedication, and creative ideas of school nurses everywhere are reflected throughout this book, so much so that recognition and appreciation to everyone are impossible. However, I would especially like to thank Marcus A. Foster, Ed.D., Superintendent, who so graciously gave me permission to use the records and procedures of the Oakland Public Schools and Mrs. Thelma S. Cook, R.N., M.P.H., who made a reality out of the project that culminated in *Redirection of School Nursing Services in Culturally Deprived Neighborhoods*. The material concerning paraprofessionals in Chapter 4 is practically all a product of her hard work and conscientious endeavor as the project coordinator and later as resource nurse for the nurse technicians in the Oakland Public Schools. Mention must also be made of Mrs. Jane E. Krigin, School Nurse Emeritus, Mt. Diablo School District, Concord, California, author in her own right, for her untiring work, fresh point of view, and critical analysis; she gave me the courage to complete this book.

Sincere thanks must also be given to Mrs. Leona Waterman for her efforts in the preparation of this manuscript. Last, but not least, my appreciation to the dedicated school nurses in Oakland, who will see their hard work and ideas reflected throughout *School Nursing in Transition*.

Doris S. Bryan

CONTENTS

1

DIMENSIONS OF SCHOOL NURSING

School nursing is a highly specialized service contributing to the process of education. That it is a socially commendable, economically practical, and scientifically sound service can be well demonstrated. It must be diligently pursued through health and educational avenues to the end that positive health among all the citizenry of this country will be a reality.

The professional nurse with her experience and knowledge of the changing growth and behavioral patterns of children is in a unique position in the school setting to assist the children in acquiring health knowledge, in developing attitudes conducive to healthful living, and in meeting their needs resulting from disease, accidents, congenital defects, or psychosocial maladjustments.

Nursing provided as part of a school program for children is a direct, constructive, and effective approach to the building of a healthful and dynamic society.*

This statement from the American Nurses' Association was written several years ago, but it is probably the most notable attempt to define school nursing for present practice. These and others similar words have been stated over and over again by nurses, health educators, physicians, school personnel, and more recently by comprehensive health planners and health manpower commissioners; yet there is always the lingering doubt if this is really what is thought and felt about school nursing. Perhaps the answer will always be in limbo because conditions change with the culture and nature of society from one era to the next. This constant change makes it almost impossible to predict the needs of any one community, let alone to predict the needs of tomorrow.

School nursing is as versatile as the nurse practicing it, as full of variety as there are differing school community needs, and as creative and innovative as the individual nurse. With the multiple problems facing parents, teachers, and students, the school nurse's role is becoming more pertinent to society than ever before. The changing needs in health, education, and society itself are reflected in the nurse's changing role in the schools.

The school nurse today is giving priority to activities to assist in the development of all boys and girls socially, emotionally, mentally, and physically; and she serves all ages from preschool through college. School nurses recognize the ultimate solution to health promotion lies with the educative process; and as a result, both community and school health education are receiving priority.

---

*From Functions and qualifications for school nurses, New York, 1966, The American Nurses' Association.

1

As more and more handicapped students are being educated in the mainstream of education, it is imperative that their health and welfare be supervised at school by well-trained and qualified health personnel. Effective school health services involve the cooperation of and coordination with all pupil personnel staff and other persons involved in the health and welfare of students within the school. Effective school health services are related to the total health program within the community.

THE EMERGING ROLE OF THE SCHOOL NURSE

School nursing can no more remain static than can any other aspect of nursing practice or of education. Early in the century much of the school nurse's time was spent on efforts to control communicable disease. Today the many effective preventive measures for the control of communicable diseases constitute a springboard for numerous activities to promote positive health. This is not to say that children and youth no longer have health problems. They do, as well as their parents, their teachers, and many of the communities in which they live. The major differences that can be identified in the role of school nurses in the past two decades are related to approach and method. School nurses seem to be recognizing the indivisibility of all aspects of health. They are utilizing the epidemiological approach, which simply means a scientific study of health status that identifies factors influencing the occurrence of health problems. They are developing an orderly approach to individual health problems through assessment, intervention, and evaluation. The ultimate solution to health promotion lies with the educative process and, as a result, both community and school health education are receiving high priority. School nurses are ceasing to be providers of isolated services. They are becoming evaluators, health counselors, interpreters, consultants, and educators.

Nurses serve schools in all parts of the country. Some are employed by boards of education and devote all of their time to work with school-age children. Others are employed by departments of health and give services to the child of school age as part of a generalized public health nursing service. Regardless of where they work, by whom they are employed, or what the scope of their responsibilities is, each nurse serving the schoolchild, from the paraprofessional aide to the school nurse practitioner, should have but one objective—to give the best service possible. This best service is designed and implemented through careful evaluation of the needs of the school and community, resources available, the amount of teamwork and administrative support within the school itself, finances, and the knowledge, skill, and personality of each nurse.

> School nurses are being forced more and more to know their role, to contribute to the educational process, and to defend their position. They are frequently asked to define what is "unique" about nursing in the school to differentiate their role from other school personnel. Perhaps their uniqueness lies in four attributes not always held by other members of the school staff:
> 1. A commitment to the practice of health as a quality of living
> 2. The ability to apply nursing skills in dealing with individual health problems
> 3. The strength of the combined utilization of counseling, consultation, and teaching skills

4. The broad community health approach working through the medium of the educational institution*

SPECIALTY BUILT ON NURSING PRINCIPLES

If we assume that school nurses are unique in the school setting primarily because they are nurses, then we can turn to nursing literature and borrow some definitions and concepts of nursing that are fundamental to all nurses and apply directly to the nurse in the school.

Some definitions and concepts from nursing literature†

Nursing It is a service to individuals and to families, therefore to society. It is based upon an art and science which mold the attitudes, intellectual competencies, and technical skills of the individual nurse into the desire and ability to help people, sick or well, cope with their health needs.

Nursing science A body of scientific knowledge from the physical, biological, and social sciences that is uniquely nursing.

Nursing diagnosis Determination of the nature and extent of nursing problems presented by individual patients receiving nursing care including family reaction.

Nursing care (1) Assistance that is provided a patient when, for some reason, he cannot provide for the satisfaction of his own needs. (2) It is commensurate with the abilities and skills of the person, the nurse providing the assistance. (3) It is derived from a study of the patient's requirements for nursing care. (4) It is directed toward making the patient better able to help himself.

Nursing function A group of similar nursing activities directed toward the satisfaction of the patient's nursing care requirements. Thus, five groups of nursing functions will consist of those related specifically to each of the nursing care requirements: (1) sustenal care, (2) remedial care, (3) restorative care, (4) preventive care, and (5) promotion of health. Two additional nursing functions which related indirectly to care must also be considered: (6) Evaluation—the process of gathering information about the patient, such as vital signs, physical examinations, diagnostic tests, and any other data that would be pertinent in planning the effects of care. (7) Planning—the process of analyzing the information gathered through the evaluation procedures and developing an appropriate course of action in accordance with the patient's needs.

Nursing activity A course of action within the province of nursing which contributes directly or indirectly to the satisfaction of the patient's nursing care requirements. It may be derived from an analysis of nursing functions.

In addition to the definitions given above, Abdellah and her associates have also provided the following list of nursing skills‡:

1. Observation of health status
   Of well person

---

*Tipple, Dorothy C.: Overview of school nursing today—new dimensions in school nursing leadership, 1969, American Association for Health, Physical Education, and Recreation.

†Excerpted with minor modifications from Abdellah, Faye G., and Levine, Eugene: Better patient care through nursing research, New York, 1965, The Macmillan Co. and Abdellah, Faye G., et al.: Patient-centered approaches to nursing, New York, 1960, The Macmillan Co.

‡From Abdellah, Faye G., et al.: Patient-centered approaches to nursing, New York, 1960, The Macmillan Co.

Of patient with physical health problem
Of patient with emotional health problem

2. Skills of communication
   Verbal
   Nonverbal
   Written

3. Application of knowledge
   Physical sciences
   Biological sciences
   Social sciences
   Nursing science
   Other general education

4. Teaching of patients and families
   Spontaneous teaching
   Planned individual instruction
   Spontaneous group teaching
   Planned group teaching

5. Planning and organization of work
   Individual patient care
   Group care of patient
   Emergency or stress situation
   As a nursing team member
   As a health team member

6. Use of resource materials
   Hospital records [school records]
   Medical records
   Reference materials
   Library

7. Use of personnel resources
   Patient, family, and friends
   Medical staff
   Dietary staff [school food service]
   Technical staff
   Social service staff
   Occupational therapy staff
   Physical therapy staff
   Hospital administrative staff [school administrative staff]
   Community agency staff
   Clergy
   Other professional nurses
   Nursing auxiliary

8. Problem-solving
   Implementing plan for care
   Evaluating care given

9. Direction of work of others
   Planning
   Assigning
   Teaching
   Supervising
   Evaluating

10. Therapeutic use of the self
    Identification of own feelings
    Identification of own needs
    Establishing own goals
       Personal

      Nursing care
      Professional
    Assessment of own growth toward goals
      Use of moral and ethical values consistent with professional nursing
11. Nursing procedures
    Specific for each specialty

All of the above definitions and skills will be illustrated and expanded in detail in following chapters. The term "patient" always refers to the schoolchild, but the meaning of the term "nurse" ranges from the paraprofessional to the school nurse practitioner performing the tasks appropriate to her knowledge, skill, and experience.

LEVELS IN SCHOOL NURSING

School nurses have the most varied education and the most varied requirements and titles of any group within the nursing profession. Some states have no certification requirements for school nurses; others require a year of study beyond the baccalaureate degree. As school nurses gain more intensive programs in continuing education, we can anticipate a higher level of professional practice. The Division of Health Services of the Denver Public Schools in the 1970 to 1971 report discusses some twenty-four new projects and activities of the services program, ranging from assistance in training teacher aides to a funded cooperative training project for school nurses to become school nurse practitioners.[1]

Classification of nursing positions ranges from the age-old superintendent of nurses to consultants, coordinators, aides, assistants, professional school nurses, and the school nurse practitioner. There is a definite need for clear-cut definitions for school nursing personnel with universal nomenclature for easy reference throughout the country. The following are suggestions for classifications:

Consultant in school nursing Education is preferably at the level of a master's degree or above. She is employed by a state or county department of education or public health and responsible as a consultant in all areas of school nursing.

Director of school nursing Education is same as the consultant. She has responsibilities for a large (fifty or over) complement of nurses and auxiliary workers.

School nursing educator Employed by a college or university and possessing a master's degree or higher. The school nursing educator's primary responsibility is to teach theory and practice in school nursing.

School nursing supervisor Possesses at least a master's degree or many years of experience and provides expert assistance to the staff nurses—usually in a smaller unit of staff (thirty-five or under).

School nurse coordinator Coordinates special programs such as those for the handicapped or other special projects. Education and experience are comparable to that of the school nursing supervisor.

School nurse practitioner A regularly prepared school-community nurse who has had special education in counseling and physical evaluation procedures to assist in the management of children with physical, emotional, perceptual, and psychological disturbances.

All the above personnel should have at least three years of experience as staff nurses in full-time school nursing programs under supervision, preferably administered by boards of education.

[1]Cushman, Wesley P.: Forty-sixth annual report, 1970-71, Division of Health Services, Denver Public Schools, J. Sch. Health **42**:225, 1972.

School-community nurse The school nurse with a baccalaureate degree and additional courses in school and community health—this is the staff nurse often termed the professional school nurse. NOTE: Called "School Nurse Teacher" in New York State.

All the above are eligible for certification or credentialing.

School nurse A registered nurse in a regularly programmed course leading to a credential or certification; the school nurse should receive guidance from a school nurse supervisor, state consultant in school nursing, or a school-community nurse and be supervised by the school-community nurse.

School nurse technician A licensed vocational or practical nurse with a variety of duties in assessment, emergency care, and other activities dependent upon the school needs. The school nurse technician will work more independently and be regularly assigned to the school. Salary is on a monthly basis.

School nurse assistant An interested individual, probably at a clerical classification with at least a high school diploma, with special orientation of ongoing staff development. Works under the supervision of a school-community nurse. Salary is on a monthly basis. Ongoing special orientation to the school health program and continuing education are a *must* for this position.

Health aide Responsibilities are dependent on individual skill and talent; work is directed. Ongoing special orientation to the school health program and continuing education are also a *must* for this position. Salary is usually on an hourly basis.

Volunteers Under the supervision of the school-community nurse, interested persons who perform a variety of activities according to ability, time, and interest.

Classifications and qualifications. The classification of school nursing power may be represented in step form. The steps start with the volunteer, the neighborhood health worker, and progress to the top step as the school nurse administrator, educator, and consultant. Detailed descriptions of the school-community nurse, the

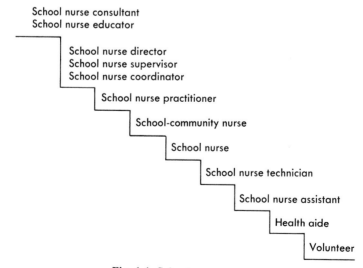

Fig. 1-1. School nurse power.

school nurse practitioner, and nurse administrator are discussed in other chapters (Fig. 1-1).

All of the above jobs could be filled by either male or female nurses serving pupils from preschool through high school.

BARRIERS

Although school nurses themselves have identified their roles and believe they are an integral and vital part of the nursing input to society today, several factors must be mentioned as deterrents to a generally assumed stable, established nursing specialty.

1. Professional school nurses are among the highest educationally prepared of all nurse specialties and have demonstrated less mobility and more job satisfaction than most other nursing groups. However, they are often stereotyped as a group that have "easy jobs" with "no challenge." This censorship comes primarily from within the profession. New graduates from nursing schools are often counseled to go into other specialties, and it is evident some nursing educators are not aware of the extent of the role and responsibilities of the school nurse.

2. Many applicants for school nursing positions are uninformed about school nursing practice and will state they would like a job in the school so they may have the same hours and vacation as the schoolchildren, little realizing that much of the school nurse's work is done before and after school hours with parents, teachers, and community groups and that there is a specific body of knowledge solely applicable to school nursing.

3. School administrators often see the nurse only as giving first aid. They are reluctant to allow the nurse to leave the school for fear that an accident may occur or sudden illness may develop. They fail to see the potentials of these highly educated specialists, not realizing the high cost of such on-the-spot service or of waste of manpower for such elementary tasks.

4. As in all professional groups, a few school nurses perpetuate the stereotype of school nursing as an "easy job." They emphatically believe "the old ways are good enough." They feel threatened by the introduction of new ideas, new methods, and new personnel.

5. Health education is a discipline that has not quite arrived and is just off the mainstream of American education, and yet this is an important aspect of school nursing. The education establishments of the United States have not shopped for or, for that matter, *had* to buy a new model of health education. The old model of "personal hygiene" has not always been used well so that today in many instances teaching hygiene is almost too easy to junk, especially when there are not enough class hours in the school day.

Health-related crisis conditions have not fully developed in our communities to add academic respectability and acceptability to health education; that is, there is not yet a driving "felt need" on the part of many educators for health education.

6. Because most schools are reacting institutions that respond to cultural needs and resources—usually belatedly and hesitatingly—significant attention, time, and money have not been provided for modern school health programs. School super-

intendents are caught up by many educational issues, pressures, controversies, and battles and endeavor to maintain school programs consistent with the consensus of professional and community thought, locally and nationally. Realistically and practically, it is the exceptional school administrator who is in a position to exert leadership to the point of influencing the nature of educational change in advance of crisis, that is, before most people in and out of schools recognize the need in the form of growing societal problems. With the problems in the field of abuse of drugs and the controversy over sex education, perhaps these crises will bring change.

SUMMARY MODEL

The dimensions of school nursing as a nursing specialty include workable definitions, recognition of barriers to good practice, and perhaps a workable philosophy. Martha Luna, staff nurse in the Oakland Public Schools, made the following statement to a group of nurses in Idaho at a school nurse workshop*:

> Now I would like to briefly describe my program as a school nurse. I was assigned this last year to three elementary schools with a total enrollment of over 2,000 pupils. These schools included two educationally handicapped classes, two educable mentally retarded classes, and one gifted class—grades kindergarten through sixth.
> I have three basic philosophies underlying my practice of school nursing:
> 1. Each pupil is a person, a unique individual of infinite worth and worthy of respect—no matter what.
> 2. Health is essential to learning.
> 3. School nursing services are indispensable to quality education and to equal opportunity for all pupils.
> The functions of school nurses are to assess, plan, implement, evaluate, study, and do research. The major portion of my time is spent on direct child care, appraisal and follow-up, and personnel conferences. Follow-up mainly includes parent contacts, referrals for care, and supervision of known health defects. I use records for *communication;* I don't do records "just to do records." Records provide transfer of information, are a history of the health of a pupil, and are a tool to expedite services.
> I am in a continual process of determining *priorities.* It seems to me that the expression "health of the school child" means "*health education* of the school child." I do think that health education is an integral part of the school health program and of the entire school curriculum. We find needs; we seek correction of defects and restoration of health; then we educate to prevent illness and to promote heath. But if we face reality, we are probably not going to change the health status or health behavior of all pupils; and there will still be illness, handicaps, and health needs to be met. I am inclined to think that the role of health personnel in the school may need to be either *health worker* or *health consultant.* The *health worker* (similar to social case worker) would provide health services including: case work, maintenance of health levels by supervision of medical and dental care, immunization levels, health history, health appraisal, and follow-up for correction of health defects. The *health consultant* (similar to guidance consultant) would promote and coordinate health education, serve as a health resource person to educators, and supplement and support the classroom teacher in health instruction. Either we do health services or we do not do health services. A little

---

*From Luna, Martha: School nursing—the way it is, presentation given at Idaho School Nurse Workshop, July, 1970.

is not enough and wastes time, effort, and money. There must be intensive involvement in health services to be effective, to actually improve the health of school children. I think that the nurse has the basic responsibility to give health services, to do those things that no one else in the school is qualified to do, those services that have medical-nursing implications. The teacher has the basic responsibility for health instruction with assistance from a nurse. The parent has the basic responsibility for obtaining medical and dental health care. The pupil has the basic responsibility for his health practices.

2

SCHOOL HEALTH
A conceptual and traditional approach

One cannot understand nursing in the school setting without a short overview of school health concepts and the traditional framework for health services. The public school in America is primarily a social institution financed by public funds to educate its youth. The health of schoolchildren is incidental in schools. Services were first instituted about seventy years ago to keep children in school by cutting down on the incidence of communicable diseases. At present, services have expanded to primary prevention of health problems through early detection and correction of health defects. These services are still maintained because it has been found that absenteeism is reduced and children, perhaps, learn easier when they are in sound mental, physical, emotional, and social health. Health instruction is now paramount in modern school health programs.

SCHOOL HEALTH CONCEPTS

There are four concepts that are basic in school health: educational, community, people, and time.

Educational concept. The fundamental purpose of the school is to educate the child. All activities including health services must be educational in nature. Examples of how the education concept functions are as follows:

1. The educational objective gives the teacher's role a more effective goal.
2. The educational aim makes the child's learning easier by providing purpose and understanding.
3. Health education must be directed toward growth and development and toward affecting attitudes and habits.

Community concept. The school health program cannot exist in isolation; it must reflect the needs and resources of the community. The school nurse works as much in the community as in the school as a liaison and interpreter. For example, the following societal concerns should be recognized and integrated into a school health program:

1. The socioeconomic needs or activities pertaining to self-preservation and earning a living
2. The community resources and activities of social and political relationships
3. The health services concerned with raising a family and activities for leisure time

The people concept. Programs are effective only as people engage in them and

10

work constructively together in a thinking, creative way. Working with others is not new. The first school health teams consisted of nurses and medical doctors; then the nurses worked with physical education teachers and added health instruction to the curriculum. At present the school health program includes the school nurse as part of the pupil-personnel team. The modern trend is to also work with the non-professional assistants in the school health program. A good health program entails a good working relationship between the school and the community, but this is not always possible; for example:

1. Working with others is not always easy because of personality conflicts, cultural differences, or gaps in educational background.
2. People may be reluctant, afraid, or hold to past practices and are thus unable to cooperate or be flexible to changes. ("We've always done it this way.")

Time concept. An effective school health program is one that is dynamic and moving forward. It is a program of multiple health activities going on today, built on the programs of yesterday, and planning for tomorrow. It is progressive in nature and expresses constructive attitudes, for example:

1. Change in expectations of administration
2. Optimum use of the school nurse's time with innovation
3. "If we don't catch up, it will surely catch up with us"

THE SCHOOL HEALTH FRAMEWORK

Traditionally the school health program has been divided into three groups of activities: healthful school living, school health services, and school health instruction. The school nurse has responsibilities in all of these activities but is by no means restricted by rigid lines of classification. The major effort of the school is pointed in one direction, and that is toward the educational programs and development of the child. The following description may provide a more precise understanding of the traditional school health program.

Healthful school living. The concept of healthful school living includes both the physical and the social environment of the school and the effect on the total health of the pupil. The school provides limitless dynamic environmental situations through which physical, social, and mental development is gained. Contributing factors to healthful school living include the following:

1. A planned program that takes into account the physical and mental health of the staff members involved in the school
2. A daily schedule of school activities best suited to the maturity and capability of each child
3. A wholesome, clean, and safe school and classroom environment with suitable lighting and color, seating, heating, ventilation, furniture, and equipment
4. Provisions for physical education with recognition of the educational and health values
5. A planned food service program that can be a laboratory for good nutrition

School health services. The program of school health services includes a number of procedures that concern the present health condition of the child, his improvement, adjustment, and protection. These procedures include the following:

1. Health appraisal that determines health status by observation; by health history; by screening tests; by medical, dental, and psychological examination;

and by measurement of height, weight, and posture (Often health appraisal will be done in a team fashion.)

2. Health counseling and follow-through that provides guidance to pupils and parents in securing care
3. Safety and emergency care procedures that provide protection from injury and care in case of accident or sudden illness, immediate first aid and notification of parents, and getting the injured or ill child home or to the hospital
4. Communicable disease control and sanitation that emphasize immunization, exclusion and readmittance, and attendance at school
5. Adjustment to individual pupil needs that demands a challenging, flexible school program aided by discerning, understanding teachers; application and knowledge of maturation of children, their growth and development, and behavioral characteristics

School health and safety instruction. Health instruction consists largely of planned learning experiences designed to influence knowledge, habits, attitudes, and conduct in regard to health and accident prevention. Health instruction may be organized utilizing a variety of approaches.

1. Direct instruction—classroom teaching, usually involving a group of pupils, a teacher, a definite time and place, and a planned sequence of learning activities
2. Integrating health topics into other school subjects—numerous opportunities available for inclusion of health concepts in the high school curriculum, but a separate health class seems to be gaining favor (Educators are recognizing that the health aspect may become lost in biological science, home economics, or social studies classes.)
3. Special activities in the school day—taking advantage of assembly programs, lectures, films, plays, the lunch program, and special projects
4. Individual health guidance—may occur at any time of the day; may result from behavior problems, medical or dental examinations, and other health appraisal findings (Any member of the staff may find himself involved in health guidance.)

The health instruction that can be covered in the secondary education program is very broad. It can include science and disease, food and nutrition, physical fitness, personal appearance, the human senses, consumer education, living safely, public health, guides to effective living in the social area, alcohol, drugs, and sex education and family life as examples ad infinitum.

PUBLIC CONCERN AND SUPPORT

If the schools are to provide adequate health programs, the public must assign such programs in high priority and let this be known to those in charge of the public schools. Along with the assignment of priority must come adequate funds to properly finance such programs.

From the time of Horace Mann, through the *Seven Cardinal Principles of Education in 1918,* the Educational Policies Commission's "The Purposes of Education in American Democracy" (1938), to the present *Imperatives in Education* by the American Association of School Administrators, health has been, and continues to be, identified as a prime objective of education. Philosophers, poets, and educators have put this into essays, poems, and position papers. Public schools pay lip service to this educational goal and believe it when they say it. But beyond generally providing a healthful and relatively safe school environment and a collection of selected health services, public schools have not committed themselves to sound programs of health and health instruction.

For all the vocal approval of health as an educational aim, public schools have, over the years, been "academically oriented" to the point of largely successfully ignoring "simple simon" health classes. Inadequate and mediocre health education programs unfortunately continue to exist in too many schools for lack of administrative support to ensure ample staffing of *well-qualified* and *interested* teachers and favorable class scheduling. Poor health instruction has been perpetuated in part because of misunderstanding, indifference, and neglect in schools—if it is offered at all. This is certainly true of other subject matter areas, of course, but perhaps to a greater extent with a relatively new field such as health education.

However, if health education has not reached academic maturity to date, it is now surely entering its adolescence. The fantastic growth of the health and medical sciences and the alarming rise in incidence of health-related societal problems, which are essentially social, economic, and political problems, guarantee it.

In the near future neither society nor public schools will be able to afford to ignore the benefits, financial and human, of health education programs in schools and communities. The essential question now is whether educators will take the bold steps necessary to meet the varied emerging health needs of our citizens and society. How much more costly the rehabilitative efforts will be if schools and communities do not act forthrightly and courageously in the establishment of comprehensive, planned health programs to help prevent illness, pain, incapacitation, and premature death. Education does not solve all the problems of living and dying, but more often than not it is the best answer available.

SUMMARY MODEL
Guidelines for a school health program

Organization for school health services will vary according to state legislation, the size of the school, available resources in personnel and equipment, and administrative provisions.

- School health services are planned as an integral part of the school educational program.
- School health services are designed to meet the needs of the specific school population.
- School health services are coordinated with the community health program.
- School health services include appraisal of the health status of students.
- School health services include appraisal of the health of school personnel.
- School health services include the interpretation of health status of students to themselves, their parents, and others who should be concerned.
- The correction of remediable defects is a major activity of the school health program.

- School health services offer assistance in the identification and education of handicapped students including those who are mentally retarded or emotionally disturbed.
- In the prevention and control of disease the school health service program carries out procedures recommended by the community health department.
- School health service personnel and instructional staff members regard the school health program as a cooperative undertaking.
- The functions and responsibilities of teachers, administrators, and other school personnel are clearly defined and understood.
- School health services in elementary and secondary schools are coordinated to provide continuous aid to the growth and development of pupils and to the protection and improvement of their health.
- School health services have been planned cooperatively and periodically evaluated by representative members of the school staff, parents, and the community.
- There are school-sponsored meetings with parents, personnel of the health department, and representatives of interested community groups and of medical and dental societies to consider the school health program and to interpret its procedures and purposes.
- The policies and procedures of the school health services program are in written form.
- There are written policies outlining procedures for emergency care and sudden illness.
- A staff member has been delegated responsibility for coordination of the school health services program within the school.
- The aims and purposes of the school health services program are interpreted to students, parents, and the community at large.
- There are planned procedures for periodic evaluation of the school health services.
- In-service provisions are made for periodic review of duties and responsibilities in school health services.

Questions for evaluation

- How adequate is the school staff's concept of the purposes of the school health services program?
- How extensive are the provisions for school health services?
- To what extent are the school health services coordinated with community health objectives?

3

THE PROFESSIONAL SCHOOL NURSE
The school-community nurse

The effectiveness of a school health program is contingent upon the competency of the school nurse and the framework in which the nurse works. Methods of accomplishing the objectives of a health program are as varied as the problems presented. However, the nurse always assumes a unique position in the school as an educator and as a clinician and nurse practitioner. Throughout the years various publications, primarily from professional organizations, have listed about 200 functions for school nurses. Vague terms and descriptions such as "administers," "coordinates with others," "confers," or "is responsible for" are usually stated and are followed by a mass of professional jargon and verbiage. These lists were important and noteworthy, and I was responsible for more than one of this type of publication. School nursing grew like Topsy, and procedures and practices often relied on one judgment or a successful practice in one area of the country.

School nursing is now coming into its own with an ever increasing, ever growing body of scientifically sound knowledge based on research from which to build programs or to redirect programs.

- From Dolores Basco's studies in Baltimore and New Jersey, high-risk groups of children can be identified so that efforts can be directed to selected youngsters rather than try to "reach" total school populations.
- In Congers, Georgia, the school nurse was working closely with the school psychologist, speech therapist, school physician, and school counselor in a team effort in a district center rather than in individual schools.
- In Oakland, California, emphasis is on parent involvement, and the school health office is developing into a center where parents telephone or come in for advice for all sorts of problems as well as health.
- Nurses in the junior and senior high schools are participating in pregnancy testing programs.
- More and more prescription drugs are being administered at schools by following carefully developed procedures.
- In Denver, Colorado, school nurses are taking on many new roles and responsibilities in their "Nurse in Expanding Roles" programs.
- With the use of nonprofessionals in many school districts, school nurses can be relieved of their many "mickey mouse" activities to practice their profession as nurses, health educators, and counselors.
- In Los Angeles, California, Joy Cauffman has made three outstanding studies in

school health. In one study she documented that any two different types of referrals (notes, telephone, parent contacts, home visits, etc.) from any two different persons (nurse, teacher, physician, principal, psychologist) had more satisfactory results in terms of nurse time, money, and outcomes.

• There is evidence of successful utilization of school nurses in group study groups, "rap sessions," if you will, with parents or students or both.

Highly developed and all-inclusive health screening programs are also being practiced in several school districts. Documentation of these programs indicates a meaningful contribution to the educational process as well as bringing valuable information to parents and the medical and dental community. Medi-screening includes physical appraisal, blood and urine examinations, speech, psychological testing, educational aptitudes, nutritional assessment, and health history and in some instances serves children from birth to age 21. These programs, of course, include a sound program for follow-up and correction of defects.

ACTIVITIES OF THE SCHOOL NURSE

The school nurse is a member of the educational team whose goal is to see that each child is in the best possible physical and emotional condition to benefit from his school experience and to reach his education objectives. The school nurse works with parents and other community workers to bridge the gap between the school and the home and various health resources in the community from preschool through college.

A nonprofessional worker is provided in some schools to assist the nurse. This worker is trained and supervised by the school nurse to perform the following duties: minor first aid, the initial vision screening, checking on immunizations, attendance problems, and transporting ill or injured children to their homes. The nonprofessional worker's services release the school nurse to work more intensively with children and parents having special health needs.

Health appraisals of all students. The nurse is responsible for obtaining health inventories or reports from parents to detect students who may have problems that need to be understood by the school staff. Some students may need guidance in obtaining adequate medical care, and the nurse is often responsible for promoting health examinations by the family's physician. Screening surveys for common defects such as vision, hearing, scalp ringworm, and heart defects; tuberculin testing; and dental inspections are done on all pupils in selected grades. Some schools continue to periodically weigh and measure pupils, but this practice is time consuming and some authorities feel it has little value. However, observations by teachers and parents remain an important facet of the appraisal process.

Assistance to students with defects. The most important contribution that the school nurse makes is to confer with students, parents, teachers, physicians and dentists, and other community agencies about students with defects. She records and reports defects and problems for the benefit of others in the school program.

Students in special education programs. The physical problems and prospects of correction are carefully examined for all students receiving special educational services.

Health supervision in school hours. The school nurse gives first aid and advice for the sick and injured as well as supervision until the parents can be contacted and the child returned home. She is also responsible for the supervision of safety practices on the school grounds and inspection for communicable diseases as well as supervision of the regulations for the control of these diseases.

Health instruction. Health instruction is a planned program based on principles of learning that takes into consideration individual differences. The school nurses, with their training and knowledge of the particular needs of the community, can be of assistance to teachers. Nurses can provide a team approach that can utilize formal classroom teaching, planning laboratory experiments, or surveying and analyzing of a health problem. Part of the nurse's activity is to coordinate supporting materials such as films, books, pamphlets, posters, and resource personnel, but this coordination is often performed by the paraprofessional.

Community health responsibilities. It is said that no knowledge is complete until it is understood enough to be applied. The health instruction of students will consequently directly affect the health status of a community. Since the school is a part of a community enterprise, the nurse's activities are involved in exchange of information with appropriate persons or agencies. The nurse participates on many committees to develop and carry out cooperative health and welfare programs.

Student school nurses. A school nurse's responsibility involves supervising the educational experience of student nurses who may be assigned to schools for field experience. Students from local colleges or universities or from other health-related agencies are sent to schools for a period of observation and practice. Some states require a set number of hours of field experience for qualification as a school nurse; time varies from a few hours to an entire college semester. Students and visitors from foreign countries may also visit the school to observe.

Reports, evaluation studies, and research. The school nurse may be involved in research and health promotion activities, and specific programs within the nursing services may be selected for evaluation. Surveys point out the need for proper programs, and after new programs are initiated, these programs need to be studied and evaluated. The findings of studies of local, current interest are shared with other departments or agencies. The accomplishments and effectiveness of the World Health Organization provide encouragement and confirmation that research and health promotion are of value; the welfare of a society is the concern of the individual nurse both on a local and worldwide basis.

PREPARATION OF THE PROFESSIONAL SCHOOL NURSE
Preservice education

School nursing is a nursing specialty that includes a sound preservice or undergraduate education leading to a baccalaureate degree and certification as a registered nurse. Yet nurses are first individuals in a society and must achieve an awareness of themselves and the world about them. They should learn how to achieve and maintain a state of mental and physical health. They must acquire effective communication habits and skills. They should develop satisfying recreational interests and skills. In addition to a liberal education, they need a very specialized education in nursing, which should include the wide gamut of sickness and health, therapy and rehabilitation, normal and abnormal behavior, anatomy and physiology, growth and development, pediatrics and geriatrics, obstetrics and surgery, body chemistry and nutrition, and physiotherapy and occupational therapy. Nurses should reinforce academic preparation with strong clinical experience to enable them to make decisions with assurance when called upon to make independent nursing judgments.

Included in the baccalaureate program or supplemented in postgraduate study, the school nurse needs knowledge in depth and practical application in the following areas of content:

1. Community nursing
2. Mental health
3. School administration
4. Theory of education and learning
5. Advanced pediatric nursing
6. Public school curriculum
7. Counseling and guidance
8. Use of audiovisual materials
9. Theory and practicum in school nursing (including vision and hearing screening)
10. Health education

With adequate preservice education, nurses will have attained the skills necessary for school nursing. They will have acquired a body of knowledge that will enable them to take their place as members of a profession. They will be able to share their knowledge with persons who differ widely from them in skills, interests, and concerns. They should then achieve this role and enact it competently. They will possess a body of knowledge that will enable them to make decisions and assume responsibility with complete awareness of the moral, legal, and ethical implications. They will truly be school-community nurses.

The content of preservice education has created great concern among all segments of the nursing profession. Content will continue to be a matter of discussion, evaluation, research, and controversy.

Continuing education

As with any professional person in this fast-moving age, continuing education is a must. Knowledge is outdated within a few years. This is particularly important for school nurses who often work alone or with very small groups of peers. They *must* assume responsibility for their own professional growth; they *must* support professional research; they *must* participate actively in professional organizations; they *must* participate in evaluation and progression of their profession; they *must* be dedicated to the welfare of their fellowmen; and they *must* recognize and respect the dignity of the individual and the sacredness of the family.

Core curriculum for school nurses

A conference on "Educational Preparation of the Nurse for School Health Work" was held in March of 1967 with funds from the United States Children's Bureau; national and state agencies sent representatives who were concerned with nursing. Specifically, representatives from boards of education, departments of health, state departments of education and health, different educational divisions of universities, and national agencies concerned with nursing attended the conference. Two points emerged as the conference progressed:

1. Commonalities of preparation in maternal and child health nursing, public health nursing, and school nursing need to be clarified and this preparation should be at the graduate level.
2. A common core of preparation for pupil personnel services should include representation from fields of medicine, psychology, guidance, social work, and related disciplines for collaboration.

The trend indicates that the professional school nurse will move toward graduate preparation that will include maternal and child health nursing and public health nursing. Preparation will also include mental aspects of nursing and learning represented under pupil personnel services.[1]

SCHOOL NURSE SPECIALIST

With additional theory and clinical experience, the present role of the school-community nurse is being expanded to provide more effective health care for the school-age child. The practitioners will be trained to give an in-depth physical assessment, health history, and evaluation of laboratory data. Their work will require initiative and judgment as well as skill to identify, prevent, refer, and follow-up health problems. They will have the ability to interpret the school needs to the community planning groups and be able to interact with pupils, family, and school staff. The nurse specialist will be able to assess religious, cultural, and socioeconomic factors influencing the family and individual health practices.

At the end of the training program the school nurse specialist will be prepared to:

1. Offer comprehensive well-child care to identify and assess the factors that may operate to produce learning disorders, psychoeducational problems, perceptive-cognitive difficulties, and behavior problems as well as those causing physical disease. The health appraisal will include the following: (a) comprehensive health history; (b) physical examination utilizing the skills of observation, palpation, percussion, and auscultation; and (c) evaluation of laboratory data (complete blood count, blood chemistry, and urine analysis).
2. Educate the school community to observe and detect health problems and assist them to integrate health concepts and principles into the curriculum.
3. Assess religious and cultural factors that may influence family and individual health practices and assimiliate these factors into the health care plan.
4. Work collaboratively with school personnel and parents to enhance the physical, mental, and social health of the school-age child.
5. Work collaboratively with other health care providers and social services in the community to ensure continuity of care.
6. Interpret school health needs to community planning.

---

[1]Stobo, Elizabeth C.: Trend in the preparation and qualifications of school nurses, presented at joint session of the American School Health Association and the American Public Health Association, School Health Section, Miami, Fla., October, 1967.

Certification, licensure, and credentialing

The nurse in the school health program carries out her role within the framework of education. Standards should be established by the state education agency for the preparation of nurses employed by boards of education. School nurses then are requested to meet these educational requirements in the form of certification standards.

Certification. Certification is evidence of completion of an individual's professional preparation for satisfactory performance in a specialized field. It is a legal procedure that authorizes the individual, upon completion of specific requirements, to perform certain services in the schools.

Licensure. Certification must be distinguished from licensure. The practitioner has met the *minimum* legal requirements established by that state and is registered to practice there by being licensed. Certification assures the public that licensed professional nurses have completed additional requirements for practice in schools. Although certification is not the only control on quality education, it does have significant influence on the preparation and selection of school personnel.

Credentialing. The school nurse who obtains the basic education in professional nursing by completing a baccalaureate degree in nursing may be eligible for a credential in school nursing. In several states nurses now take up to an additional year of graduate study before being eligible for a school nurse credential. Courses usually include work in depth in child growth and development, mental health, curriculum development, advanced pediatrics, and health education methods and media.

Staff development education

What is staff development? The school nursing staff should participate in regularly scheduled professional education sessions. Community specialists or guest speakers may be invited to participate in these professional sessions, or small study groups may be organized to pursue and develop new policies and procedures.

School nurses participate in orientation of teachers and parent groups to current aspects of public health at school meetings or conferences. Attendance at workshops and professional conferences is encouraged. They also participate in school in-service training for total school personnel.

Graduate education. Graduate education in school nursing admits a school nurse to a master's degree program that encompasses a broad foundation in education, behavioral sciences, and the field of specialization.

Continuing education. School nurses often enter a varied program for professional and personal growth to qualify for opportunities for promotion for supervision, consultation, administration, and university teaching. All such positions demand additional preparation through continuing education.

SCHOOL HEALTH PROGRAMS AND
SCHOOL NURSE ACTIVITIES IN TRANSITION

Leaving the traditional framework for school health programs and making the transition into the future, we find that the school still reflects the needs and resources of the community. School nurses are faced with problems our culture has only fairly recently recognized as such, as illustrated in the following list:

1. Children do not value performance of chores as a means of earning the

privilege. Monetary allowances are too free; the value of earning money through effort expended is lacking.

2. There is greater mobility than heretofore via the automobile. This freedom has created problems of promiscuity and venereal disease.

3. The need for more than one job in families to keep up with extravagance requires mothers as well as fathers to work outside the home, thus spending less time with the children. There is less sense of belonging or pride in one's heritage. Parents may provide materially even to excess but brush aside love and caring.

4. The mobility trend in America has caused suburban youth to become an impersonal part of clubs and organizations; mobility has created employment problems for men and insecurity for children.

5. Automation and computerized programming create a sense of depersonalization and may produce a statistic instead of a creative, thinking human being. The zest for learning needs to be turned from decision making for children to decision making *with* children.

6. Children have more leisure time and decreased means of spending this time in worthwhile activities. The advertising on television emphasizes materialistic life and threatens the socioeconomic level of families. People live from day to day with monetary satisfaction unable to feel security and to plan ahead.

7. Children of broken homes have experienced physical or emotional abuse from the mother or father or both. The one-parent family with the mother taking on the father's role has frustrated husband and sons.

8. Children are greatly influenced by adult example as they see the use of alcohol, tobacco, and drugs. Drugs and tranquilizers have become an escape for tensions of living and may be used for attempted suicide.

9. Children are growing up in an overpopulated country and are faced with undersanding problems of survival of man. Safety hazards of rapid transit and overcrowded highways along with the health hazards of air, water, and noise pollution influence our life today.

10. Problems of mental illness, child abuse, moral decay, promiscuity, illegitimacy, perversion, and venereal disease are some of the stresses of modern life.

It is evident that the school nurse's role today goes beyond working with the classroom teacher, parent, school physician, and students. Today school nurses are expected to make judgments and professional decisions that they share with guidance counselors, psychologists, and special teaching personnel of the visually, speech, or auditorially handicapped and the retarded or emotionally disturbed. It is essential for the school nurse to understand normal growth and development and the clinical deviations from a medical viewpoint. Nurses must also understand deviations of learning from an educator's viewpoint.

Definition of professional responsibility

To meet the challenge of education school nurses must become life-long members of a professional health team. Since there is no one way of viewing a health problem, an interdisciplinary approach is needed. In this transitory age it will be the responsible nurse who will effect mature decisions. The nurse will be that versatile, adaptable kind of a person who is able to communicate and interpret knowledge.

The nurse holds fast to the understanding of human values as presented by the philosophical statements of Dr. Harold Lasswell, Carl Rogers, and Abraham Maslow.[2] The nurse will be flexible and know the importance of participation, motivation, reinforcement, and enrichment. Although computers may gather data, facts alone will not solve health problems or produce responsible citizens.

SUMMARY MODEL

Here are a few questions nurses need to ask themselves. The answers are self-evident. If these questions cannot be answered correctly, why not? How can one go about getting an appropriate answer?

1. How much are you attached to the local power figure? Are you a "Yes Sir"– "No Sir" person? Consider what you can contribute from two professions. Do you work *with* educators or *for* the administration?
2. Are you a pretender to the classroom teacher? Not a resource person or a health expert but a nurse teaching health to *all* grades with little preparation or skill. Teachers are not qualified to do this; then why the school nurses?
3. Are you an expediter of screening programs? Is not your background education and experience as a nurse more complex than a knowing how to use a scale, an audiometer, and the various positions of the illiterate E?
4. Do you provide jitney service for lonesome or sick children? This means you have a car, insurance, and have the ability to drive.
5. Do you waste time driving from one school to another to "cover" both for a half day?
6. Can you work any place? Need no privacy or a pleasant place to work? If what you do is meaningful or relevant, you need the setting to work as efficiently as possible.
7. Are you a paper shuffler and a clerical worker?
8. Are you a truant officer? Why have a clerk do this when the nurse is around!
9. Are you a "miracle worker" setting up a whole school health program by yourself with no involvement with school, community, or parents?
10. Are you a first aider?—Don't teach anyone else to assume these duties, just call wherever the nurse is!
11. Are you your own medical director rather than a nursing director?
12. Are you paid as a professional within the school? If you perform as a professional, you should be paid as a professional.
13. Are school nurses getting all children into the mainstream of complete health care? Are you helping children and parents know what to expect when they are referred to a medical or dental resource? Do parents understand the concept of comprehensive health care?
14. Are you teaching health education so that children and parents know how to promote health and prevent diseases?
15. How are your communications with the medical community and the school administration?
16. Are you, as the school nurse, an integral part of the team in evaluation or assessment of children?

---

[2]Murphy, Maribeth L.: Values and health problems, J. Sch. Health **43**:23, 1973.

4

PARAPROFESSIONAL SCHOOL HEALTH WORKERS

One of the major problems of education today is how to educate children who are essentially the product of socioeconomic change in the United States. Population changes have imposed new demands on the community's institutions and created many problems of adjustment between man and his environment and between man and man. The increased technical nature of the health program has made great demands upon professional time. There is a need to utilize the abilities and skills of a variety of school nurses to greater advantage.

DETERMINATION AND ASSIGNMENT OF DUTIES

Determination of the duties of the various paraprofessionals is essential in order to select the right person for the position. Likewise, school nurses need to know how these workers function; and the school personnel must be oriented to activities that can be performed by health assistants:

1. There must be a clear distinction between professional and the nonprofessional tasks.
2. There must be development of a job description for the nonprofessional personnel. This is done on the basis of what persons can do, not on what the nurses feel they would like to give up.
3. Careful selection and training of personnel is imperative.
4. Continuous supervision by professional staff, trained to supervise, is necessary.
5. Preparation of school and nursing staff for acceptance and utilization of the paraprofessional.
6. There must be a continuing evaluation of the effectiveness of such assistance.*

The functions of the school nurse have not only changed but have greatly expanded as well. In establishing guidelines for the auxiliary worker or health aide, nonprofessional tasks are those not requiring professional skill or judgment. However, it is the responsibility of the personnel department of a school district to prepare a description of the position, the purpose of the classification, the major duties, and the distinguishing features.

---

*From Bryan, Doris S.: School nurse assistants—new dimensions in school nursing leadership, Washington, D. C., 1969, American Association for Health, Physical Education, and Recreation.

Redirection of school nursing activities[1]

One of the earliest programs on the use of the paraprofessional personnel began in Oakland, California, in 1965 as a part of a nursing study, and since that time the number of paraprofessionals has grown from three to twenty-seven in five years and is increasing each year.

The paraprofessional is assigned to work in a school under the supervision of the school nurse and the direction of the principal. The paraprofessional acts as an assistant to the nurse by performing a variety of selected tasks for which the paraprofessional can quickly be trained. The major purposes for the incorporation of these workers into the health program are as follows:

1. To provide better nursing coverage to schools, particularly the large schools and schools located in areas of great need.
2. To release the school nurse from the time-consuming routine tasks of the health office—the care of minor illness, maintenance of health records, immunization assessment and follow-up, and so forth. By releasing nurses from these routine duties, nurses are allowed to spend their time working with children who have more serious health problems and unmet health needs and in special health programs.

Many school districts across the country now utilize the services of the paraprofessional. Thelma S. Cook and I published the following report describing how paraprofessionals could be incorporated into a health service program in *The Journal of School Health**:

> The project, "Redirection of School Nursing Services in Culturally Deprived Neighborhoods," grew out of two major concerns confronting the Department of Health Services of the Oakland Public Schools:
> 1. Developing more effective ways for the school nurse to cope with the problems of the culturally and educationally disadvantaged child, the Oakland community being confronted with a complex of problems broadly characteristic of large metropolitan cities.
> 2. Developing more effective methods of utilizing the unique knowledge and skills of the school nurse, freeing her from such time-consuming routine burdens as record-keeping, care of minor first aid, and so on, so that she might provide a more comprehensive service to students and families with special health needs.
>
> This three-year study, approved and financed by the Children's Bureau, began May 1965 with the following three objectives:
> 1. To determine if a planned program of personal contacts by the school nurse with parents in culturally diverse areas would increase parental action toward maintenance and promotion of the schoolchild's health and the prevention of illness.
> 2. To determine if non–nurse assistants could release a school nurse by carrying out, under supervision, selected routine nursing functions.
> 3. To determine if released time for a school nurse would be, in fact, used for the exercise of higher nursing knowledge and skills.

---

*Excerpted with minor modifications from Bryan, Doris S., and Cook, Thelma S.: Redirection of school nursing services in culturally deprived neighborhoods, J. Sch. Health **39**:247, 1969.

[1]Bryan, Doris, and Cook, Thelma S.: Redirection of school nursing services in culturally deprived neighborhoods, final report, December, 1968, Oakland Unified School District.

The study was conducted in three experimental schools, located in low socio-economic areas and with enrollments ranging from 831 to 1,116. There were three comparable control schools.

The student sample selected to receive the more concentrated nursing service in the experimental schools consisted of approximately 1,000 kindergarten pupils with a nearly equal number of kindergartners in the control.

A full-time school nurse was assigned to each of six schools, three experimental and three control, and were matched according to education and experience. Selection of nurses for the experimental schools was also based upon their interest in participating in the project.

The job of the school nurse assistant was identified, a plan for training developed, and the three full-time positions filled with women who met the qualifications of the Oakland Public School classified position of Typist-Clerk I, the qualifications set by project personnel, and their interest in working in a new capacity in an experimental project. Each experimental school had a school nurse assistant.

The project was evaluated on the basis of whether the three objectives were achieved. Eight indicators of parent response were identified and an individual pupil record developed to collect this data for each member of the student sample, experimental and control. A time and activity study was designed and carried out by the experimental school nurses, control school nurses, and school nurse assistants for four statistical months of each of the three years of the project. A performance appraisal was developed and carried out on the school nurse assistants twice during the first year and yearly thereafter. Special reports were prepared by the experimental school nurses concerning parent study groups, participation in community activities, and health education activities for the student sample group. The individual pupil record provided for an account of all nursing service to an individual child. In addition, an evaluation conference was conducted at the termination of the project, the members of the evaluating group being experts in school health, nursing, public health, and education.

The following conclusions were reached:

1. Non-professional personnel can perform selected school nursing technical tasks efficiently and, under given circumstances, will release the school nurse, in time, for more intensive work with certain children presenting health problems that affect school progress.

2. Personal contacts by school nurses with parents in low-income neighborhoods does increase parent action in establishing an acceptance of health care and correction of health defects.

3. School nurses can give up routine tasks and can practice nursing skills with greater sophistication, more perception, and improved quality of total nursing performance. The redirection of nursing services is primarily the redirection of the nurse herself and calls for a new approach to in-service education to help the nurse identify goals of nursing service that can be realistically achieved in culturally diverse schools through nursing intervention rather than emphasis on activities to be performed or procedures to be carried out which may be unrelated to the needs and problems of students and their families. Redirection, then, is the development of a more highly skilled nurse practitioner.

Evaluation of school nurse assistants' time

Table 1 demonstrates that the school nurse assistants spend 70.44 percent of their time (averaging 5' 23" per day) during the first year, 73.32 percent (5' 38") the second year, and 71.13 percent (5' 21") the third year in performing specific routine nursing functions assigned to them. In addition to this, the school nurse

Table 1. Distribution of time* spent by school nurse assistants in performing specific services and activities assigned to them, September 1965 to February 1968

Services and activities assigned to school nurse assistant	1965-1966 school year		1966-1967 school year		1967-1968 school year	
	AVERAGE TIME PER DAY	% OF TIME PER DAY	AVERAGE TIME PER DAY	% OF TIME PER DAY	AVERAGE TIME PER DAY	% OF TIME PER DAY
Direct child care	2′ 19″	30.30	2′ 31″	32.95	2′ 23″	31.46
Service to children with attendance problems	8″	1.83	9″	1.78	15″	3.32
Health appraisal activities						
Health appraisal reports	10″	2.19	17″	3.81	4″	0.97
Initial classroom vision screening	16″	3.46	8″	1.67	–	–
Vision retest	8″	1.72	3″	0.91	7″	1.65
Audiometric screening	1″	0.28	1″	0.15	–	–
Examination by school physician	3″	0.74	–	–	–	–
Weighing and measuring	1″	0.15	2″	0.38	1″	0.15
Student records and reports	1′ 5″	14.19	1′ 8″	15.01	56″	12.31
Individual child health supervision						
Making appointment for student	1″	0.04	1″	0.02	–	–
Immunizations	10″	2.27	14″	2.99	9″	2.03
Health education activities						
Health education materials	8″	1.78	5″	1.04	6″	1.48
Bulletin boards, displays, exhibits	7″	1.54	2″	0.39	1″	0.17
Assisting nurse in educational projects	17″	3.72	25″	5.47	23″	5.18
Maintenance of nurse's office	26″	5.69	29″	6.60	51″	11.08
Maintenance of first-aid supplies in classroom	3″	0.54	3″	0.65	6″	1.33
Total	5′ 23″	70.44	5′ 38″	73.82	5′ 21″	71.13

*All computations to the nearest whole minute. No fraction of a minute shown.

assistants spend approximately 4 percent of their time in conference with the school nurse, and the school nurses spend slightly less than 5 percent of their time either in conference with or providing direct supervision to the assistants.

Job classification

The National Educational Association Department of School Nurses Commission on Standards for School Nursing Services believes that personnel staffing patterns must be developed and implemented in order to provide quality health services to schoolchildren. Further, the commission believes that nonprofessional and technical duties associated with the school health services program should be performed by the paraprofessionals under the direct supervision of the school nurse. This commission recommends guidelines for utilization of school health aides, listing the functions, qualifications, the job classification, in-service education, and the technical aspects in many areas of school nursing.

The following are examples of job classifications and in-service programs for the school nurse technician, the nurse assistant, and the health aide. An employment interview guide is included that can be helpful for persons who are not too familiar with the activities and qualifications for these positions. The guide can also be adapted for evaluations by the worker as well as for different job classifications. The material given below was developed by Thelma Cook while she was coordinator of the Nurse Assistant program in Oakland, Calif.

SCHOOL NURSE TECHNICIAN

Purpose of classification. To select the person whose responsibilities will include the following:

1. To act as an assistant to the school nurse, carrying out selected activities ordinarily done by the nurse, and to manage the health office in the absence of the nurse.
2. To perform selected individual child assessment procedures or other selected health activities that may be a part of a special project or program.
3. To set up and maintain student health records, emergency files, special project records, and other related health records as well as perform a variety of other clerical duties.

Major duties of classification. Under the supervision of the school nurse the school nurse technician does the following:

1. Manages the health office.
2. Receives all students who come to the office seeking assistance; assesses their problems; provides care for injuries and emergency illness, seeking guidance from the school nurse as may be necessary; and transports pupils home or to a source of medical care as may be indicated.
3. As may be directed by the school nurse, plans and carries out the initial vision screening tests of children in designated grades; may also participate in selected follow-up activities.
4. Sets up and maintains student health records, distributing and collecting health appraisal forms.
5. Assesses individual immunization needs of children and provides necessary follow-up.

6. Performs selected individual child assessment procedures or other selected health activities that may be a part of a special project or special health program.

7. Participates in selected health education activities, assisting the school nurse with the many detailed planning activities necessary for a successful education program.

8. As may be directed by the school nurse, may do some selected defect follow-up such as making appointments.

INTERVIEW OR EVALUATION RECORD* *School nurse technician*		
Qualifications or skills	**Score**	**Comments**
Education, experience, and job knowledge required: High school graduation with licensed vocational nurse certificate. Must have completed a probationary period of satisfactory experience in the public school setting and must have a valid American Red Cross First Aid Certificate, Multimedia System. Must have clerical skills and must own and drive a car.		
Skills required: Must be able to skillfully manage ill or injured pupils, advising both parents and teachers concerning appropriate action to be followed. Must be able to skillfully plan and carry out well-defined health activities with a minimal amount of nursing supervision. Must be able to provide a meaningful and educational observational type of experience for the new school nurse assistant I.		
Responsibility for independent action: Required to use judgment in assessing the individual needs of students who come to the health office seeking assistance and must be able to take appropriate action. Nursing supervision is minimal but always available by phone. Must be able to set up health files, obtain health reports, and carry out all clerical aspects of the health office. Must be able to plan and carry out well-defined health program activities.		
Responsibility for the direction of others: None.		
Responsibility for contacts with others: Routine contact with pupils, school personnel, clinics, physicians, other professional workers, and parents on a variety of student health problems.		

*Suggested code: Interview guide—use as checklist. Evaluation guide—satisfactory = S; needs further help = U.

9. May participate in the initial orientation of school nurse assistant by providing observational and participant-observational types of experience.

Distinguishing features. The school nurse technician may be considered the licensed practical (vocational) nurse, the "journeyman" level of the school nurse technician. Procedures are well defined, but supervision is minimal, and there is greater need for the exercise of independent judgment. The school nurse technician functions more independently and does more overall planning for health programs.

SCHOOL NURSE ASSISTANT

Purpose of classification. To select the person whose responsibilities will include the following:

1. To act as an assistant to the school nurse by performing selected duties ordinarily done by the school nurse.
2. To perform selected individual child assessment procedures or other selected health activities that may be a part of a special project or program.
3. To perform a variety of clerical duties including maintenance of student health records, completion of special project forms, and other related health records.

Major duties of classification. Under the supervision of the school nurse the school nurse assistant does the following:

1. Maintains the health office.
2. Greets all students who come to the health office seeking assistance, assesses their individual needs, and provides care as training permits or refers to the school nurse or principal as indicated.
3. Provides care for minor injury and care for emergency illness.
4. Transports sick or injured pupils home as may be necessary.
5. Assists the school nurse in performing the initial vision screening tests and may participate in selected follow-up activities.
6. Assists in the distribution and collection of health appraisal forms and related activities as may be delegated.
7. Assesses individual immunization needs of children and participates in selected follow-up activities.
8. Maintains student health records and other related records. Maintains records and reports having to do with special projects or special health programs.
9. Performs selected individual child assessment procedures or other selected health activities that may be a part of a special project or program.
10. Participates in selected health education activities such as maintenance of bulletin boards and the ordering and maintenance of health education material. Assists the school nurse in the many detailed activities necessary for a successful education program.
11. Performs clerical duties as may be assigned by the school nurse and which are consistent with those of typist-clerk I.

Distinguishing features. This classification differs from a nurse technician in that high school graduation and a typing skill are required but no health preparation is necessary. The scope of the duties is less. Procedures are well defined, there is supervision by the school nurse, and concentrated orientation or continuing education is needed.

SCHOOL HEALTH AIDE

Purpose of classification. To select the person who will be able to act as an assistant to the school nurse by performing selected tasks ordinarily done by the school nurse.

Major duties of classification. Under the supervision of the school nurse, the school health aide does the following:

1. Keeps the health office neat and attractive and in order to receive students.
2. Greets all students who come to the health office seeking assistance, assesses their individual needs, and provides care as training permits or refers to the school nurse or principal if indicated.
3. Provides care for minor injuries and minor illnesses.
4. Transports sick or injured pupils home as may be necessary.
5. Assists in the maintenance of student health records, records the results of vision screening tests, complies with the immunization or other health regulations, as may be directed by the school nurse.
6. Assists the school nurse and principal in carrying out the immunization regulations.
7. Assists in the distribution and collection of health appraisal forms.
8. Other duties as assigned by the school nurse and for which adequate training and supervision have been provided.

Distinguishing features. This classification differs from school nurse assistant in that supervision is immediately available and much less self-direction and independence are required. A typing skill is not required and the scope of duties is less. This position could be filled by a community worker who is paid on an hourly basis.

GENERAL ORIENTATION AND TRAINING OUTLINE FOR PARAPROFESSIONALS

All newly employed paraprofessionals must be provided with the orientation and training necessary to perform the duties outlined in the previous section under specific job classifications. The orientation and training program consists of three major parts:

1. Sixteen-hour basic orientation and training course (outlined below).
2. The American Red Cross Standard First Aid Course, Multimedia System. This is an eight-hour course, and an American Red Cross First Aid Certificate is issued upon satisfactory completion.
3. Observational and participant-observational experiences with a qualified school community nurse or school nurse technician, depending on need.

The basic orientation and training course is usually presented in four separate four-hour sessions as follows:

Meeting number 1 (four hours)

1. School assignment
  Source of direction for the school nurse assistant
    The school nurse
    The school principal
    The regional consultant for pupil personnel services

    The coordinator of school nurse assistant program

    The classified personnel office

2. Some general rules for the paraprofessional

    Nurses' daily report

    Mileage

3. Evaluation schedule

    Probationary period

4. Role and function of the school nurse in the school district

5. Objectives and activities of the paraprofessionals

6. Management of the sick or injured child

    First-aid tray

    "First Aid and Emergencies"

    How to take a temperature and care of thermometers

    Exclusion from school

Meeting number 2 (four hours)

1. Management of the sick or injured child (continued)

    Shock and prevention of shock

    Children with special health problems—convulsive disorders, diabetes, asthma, and so forth

    Administration of prescription drugs

    Transporting the sick or injured child home

    Emergency file

2. Vision screening

    Snellen test

    Color vision test

    Records and reports having to do with vision testing

3. Communicable disease control

    Communicable disease chart

    A manual for the control of communicable diseases

    Immunizations

Polio	Rubeola
Rubella	Tuberculin Tine test
DPT	Other

Meeting number 3 (four hours)

1. Management of the health office

    Some helpful hints for the paraprofessional

    How does the paraprofessional explain her job and identify herself?

    Answering the phone and taking messages

2. Observation of public health

    Some general signs of illness

3. The hearing program

4. Student health records and reports

    Health record form

    Defect card

Health appraisal forms
Immunization records
Other
5. Health education
Ordering health education materials
Preparation of bulletin boards

Meeting number 4 (four hours)

1. Special problems of students
Drug abuse
Dental health
Venereal disease
Sickle cell anemia
2. Review
Questions and answers
Discussion of special problems

THE FUTURE OF THE PARAPROFESSIONAL

All future expectations of the school nurse's role that respond to the strain of the environment—programs to assess learning problems, anticipate care needs, and make prognoses concerning emotional difficulties—point to the need for having school health aides. "If school nurses are to become practitioners . . ., they must become participants and contributors to the furtherance of professional education *and* nursing. . . . She must be professional nurse and professional educator."*

Jerome Lysaught believes that nurses themselves need to declare what they can do and demonstrate their capacity to do it. There seems to be plenty of opportunity for anyone interested in a health career. More than 200 health-related occupations have developed from the three basic disciplines of medicine, nursing, and dentistry.

School nurses must become skilled, knowledgeable practitioners able to make "triage" decisions—decisions dealing with channeling, management, and knowledge of alternatives to solve problems. When knowledge of the basic areas of pathology, bacteriology, physiology, anatomy, and embryology is complemented by training in new medical technology, the school nurse practitioner is making a necessary transition. This reorientation should include a development of her understanding of education and of school problems.[2]

Continuing education that will provide reorientation is needed for nurses. As nursing education has evolved, increased emphasis has been placed on values, emotions, mental health, and decision making. Many professionals believe that the focus of school health education should change from matters of physical fitness, nutrition, safety, anatomy, and disease control to the broader concern for personal development and mental health. Within this broad area, the previous subject areas could be covered, but the emphasis should be the emerging and evolving personality of the student.

---

*From Lysaught, Jerome P.: Bell, book and candle—the role of the school nurse, Today's Education, p. 24, January, 1973.
[2]Hinricks, Marie: Review of "Introduction to professions," J. Sch. Health **42:**15, 1972.

Among the ways suggested to benefit the educational program is the use of the nurse as a resource consultant. This may involve retraining to define her new role. The resource consultant may be available for in-service education for both professional and paraprofessional personnel. This new role will require expert communication and coordination skills, with a special interest and education in specific areas of school nursing practice such as screening programs.

The constructive and creative utilization of paraprofessional personnel will allow the school health nurse to respond to the demands of an expanding profession.

SUMMARY MODEL
School nurse assistant program objectives for the 1972-1973 school year

The program objectives of the school nurse assistant, working under the supervision of the school community nurse and the direction of the principal, are as follows:

1. To assist children in the resolution of minor health problems that arise during the course of the school day, giving the aid necessary to children presenting such problems in order that they may remain in school if at all possible; and, for children who are unable to remain in school because of health reasons, to arrange for their safe return home.
2. To assist the school nurse with clerical and selected technical tasks, for which adequate training and instruction have been provided, in order that the school nurse will have more time to work with children having the more serious health problems or in special health programs involving her school.

It is the belief of the school nurse assistants that, by working toward these objectives, they will be making a definite contribution toward the primary purpose of educators; that is, ". . . to provide all students served with an equal opportunity to develop to their greatest potential their particular skills, competencies, and other abilities to the end that they may become responsible and useful participants in our democratic society. . . . Assisting children in the resolution of health problems in order that they may attend class in greater physical comfort and personal security will aid the school district in the achievement of its six identified educational goals—intellectual development, responsible citizenship, vocational and economic competence, health, lifelong learning, and appreciation for natural resources."*

During the 1971-1972 school year, the school nurse assistants placed emphasis on their first objective. During the twelve-week sample period, they were able to return to class 82.02 percent of the students they served. Emphasis during the 1972-1973 school year will again be placed on this same objective.

Measurement of achievement

Achievement may be measured by obtaining the following information:
1. Number and kinds of problems managed by the nurse assistant
2. Number of students able to return to class after having been given assistance by the nurse assistant
3. Number of students for whom a safe return home or source of medical care has been arranged by the nurse assistant

---

*From unpublished material by Thelma S. Cook, Oakland, Calif.

5

SCHOOL NURSING PRACTICE
Direct child care

The concept of school nurses being concerned with only the child while he is at school should yield to the more realistic concept of the school nurse being concerned about the other people with whom the child comes in contact. School nurses are interested in improving family and community health as a whole, but their primary responsibility is the child, and it is on the child that they must focus their school nursing practice. School nurses deal directly with the child in the areas of health appraisal by preventing disease, dealing with existing health problems, and giving first-aid care in emergencies.

The procedures given in this chapter are to serve as guidelines for the nurse in these areas and are consistent with school practices throughout the country. It must be remembered that these procedures provide evidence for various nursing interventions of follow-up and correction through parents, teachers, and community help providers. Procedures should be based on up-to-date research, state and local legislation, current local practices, and community resources.

The school nurse is probably the best prepared to initiate a framework for procedures for nursing services. Approval of these policies and procedures for school nursing practice by the local medical society, the health department, and the board of education legally protects the nurse. It is from within a framework of approved procedures that nurses can implement and improve their practice.

RECORDS AND REPORTS
School health records

Health records are usually maintained for every child enrolled in school; a sample of the School Health Record form appears in Fig. 5-1. These records are included in the child's total school record, usually called his Cumulative Folder, and are kept in the classroom. Teachers and other school personnel often make notations on these records, but only pertinent data should be recorded.

Nurses commonly use rosters for class information on screening programs, physical and dental examinations, immunization status, and pertinent types of information. A Nurse's Follow-up Record form (Fig. 5-2) is usually kept in a tickler file on children with defects who need follow-up. When the defect has been corrected, these cards may be discarded.

Defect cards are invaluable to the nurse when children have permanent disabilities, since they are easily accessible to inform teachers and administrators of

Text continued on p. 42.

Name

Last   First   Middle

Birthdate   Sex

Special Notation

	R									

Health History Year

Chicken Pox

Measles (Red)

Measles (German)

Mumps

Rheumatic Fever

Heart Defect

Convulsions

T.B. Contact

Diabetes

Allergies

Frequent Colds

Ear Infection

Other (Specify)

Date

Grade

Vision Without Glasses — R 20/ L 20/

Vision With Glasses — R 20/ L 20/

Hearing — R, L

Physical Exam.

Dental Exam.

Health Inventory

Special Services

Most Recent Tests and Immunizations

Date   Comments

DPT

DT

TET

S.P.

Polio

Measles

TB Skin Test

Chest X-Ray

Urine Test

Medical or Social Agencies (name of physician, dentist) assisting family.

(Over)

(Front)

Continued.

Fig. 5-1. School Health Record.

Date	Reason for Referral	Comments	Signature

(Back)

Fig. 5-1, cont'd. For legend see p. 35.

NAME:

(LAST)   (FIRST)   BIRTH DATE:

GRADE   ROOM   ADDRESS   PHONE   SCHOOL

Date and Problem   Remarks

A

(Front)   **NURSE'S FOLLOW-UP RECORD**

Date and Problem   Remarks

B

DIVISION OF SPECIAL SERVICES — DEPARTMENT OF HEALTH SERVICES

(Back)

Continued.

Fig. 5-2. **A** and **B**, Nurse's Follow-up Record. **C** and **D**, Instructions for use of Nurse's Follow-up Record.

INSTRUCTIONS FOR USE OF NURSE'S FOLLOW-UP RECORD

_____(use pencil)_____
Name   Last   First   Address   Phone

____(use pencil)_____   ____(use pencil)____
Grade   Room   Birth Date   School

GENERAL INSTRUCTIONS:

C

1. A card will be made for every student having a health problem which requires follow-up.

2. Use flags to denote type of problem as follows:

Red – Heart	Green – Miscellaneous
Blue – Eyes	Black – Diabetes-Epilepsy
Yellow – Ears-Nose-Throat	Pink – C.C.S.
Orange – Tuberculosis	

(Front)

3. In left margin, record in red each parent contact made.

CODE		
T.C.	Telephone Call
H.V.	Home Visit
N.	Written Communication
C.	Conference at School

4. When condition has been corrected, keep card until information has been recorded on Health Record and on Annual Report.

D

5. Send card to nurse when student transfers to another Oakland school. If record is closed, card is to be filed with cumulative record.

6. Only after child has failed threshold hearing test is card initiated.

7. Comments on card should be brief.

(Back)

Fig. 5-2, cont'd. For legend see p. 37.

NURSE'S DAILY REPORT

School_____

		Health Conference						Referrals					

Scheduled Teacher—Nurse Conference

_____

_____
(Date)

_____
(Nurse)

First Aid	Student	Phone	Parent	Parent-Note	School Staff	Community Agencies	Medical	Dental	Special Services	Health Education	Meetings	Remarks

13-0148-02 20M269-6

Continued.

Fig. 5-3. A, Nurse's Daily Report. **B** and **C,** Weekly tally.

WEEKLY TALLY

Nurse/Nurse Assistant _____

Other (specify) _____

| | School | | Month | | Week Ending | |

B

	ITEM	MONDAY	TUESDAY	WEDNESDAY	THURSDAY	FRIDAY	TOTAL NUMBER
Conference	First Aid						
	Student						
	Parent - Phone						
	Other - Phone						
	Parent - School						
	Home - Visit						
	Parent Note						
	School Staff						
	Community Agency						
Referrals	Medical						
	Dental						
	Special Services						
	Student Record, etc.						
	Meetings						
Parent Initiated Contacts	Phone						
	Conference						

REMARKS: _____

_____

_____

Fig. 5-3, cont'd. For legend see p. 39.

Name _____   Date _____

INTERVIEWS: PARENT QUESTIONNAIRE		MONDAY	TUESDAY	WEDNESDAY	THURSDAY	FRIDAY	TOTAL NUMBER
Referals Completed	Medical						
	Dental						
	Other (specify)						
	Transportation Provided						
Health Screening	Project						
	Other (specify)						
	Coordinator						
	Assistant						
	Case Conference						
Health Inservice	Teacher Conference						
	Classroom						
	Small Group Pupils						
	Small Group Parents						
	School and/or Community Projects						
In-service	Leader						
	Participants						
INTERVIEWS: PARENT QUESTIONNAIRE		MONDAY	TUESDAY	WEDNESDAY	THURSDAY	FRIDAY	TOTAL NUMBER
Project Activities	Record Keeping						
	Record Review						
	Project Meetings (specify)						

REMARKS: _____

_____

Please use tally marks in appropriate squares and numbers for totals. These reports are to be filled in daily with the last entries made on Friday of each week. Place the completed form in the school mail for pick-up on Monday at your school. Send the report to Sue Perry, START Center, Room 215.

DB:klm
9/27/72

2

Fig. 5-3, cont'd. For legend see p. 39.

health problems and follow-up. These cards should be sent with other school records when pupils transfer from one school to another.

Nurses' Daily Report forms

There are as many nurse activity forms as there are school nurses and school districts. None are very good; however, the important premise is that there *is* one and it is kept up-to-date. A sample Nurses' Daily Report form is shown in Fig. 5-3.

Perhaps the school district is not concerned with the nurses' activities; however, a record of each child coming to the nurse's office and the result of the visit *must* be kept. People forget and parents and teachers are misinformed; an accurate record should be kept for easy and effective reference. This again is for the protection of the school, the child, and the nurse.

Close scrutiny of these records offers many clues for evaluation of needs, policies, programs, and reduction or reemphasis of services. These records may give the nurse or teacher new ideas for health instruction or new strategies for effective interventions.

Health memos

It is often expedient to send to teachers and other school personnel written information regarding the health status of pupils. It can confirm a casual conference and serve as a reminder or reemphasize a point for a busy teacher. The Health Memo form shown in Fig. 5-4 is a simple yet effective form for this purpose.

PROGRAM
PERIOD I IV
II V
III VI

HEALTH MEMO

TO:

RE: DATE ______

NAME ______ GRADE ______ COUNSELOR ______

Signed ______

13-0163-02 30M670—1 Title ______

Fig. 5-4. Health Memo.

AUTHORIZATION FOR INFORMATION

I hereby authorize

Hospital _____

Physician _____

Address _____ Telephone _____

to give any or all information contained in the record of:

_____
Name   Birth date

_____
Medical Record Number

to the Oakland Public Schools, Health Services, 1025 Second Avenue, Oakland, California 94606.

_____
(Signature of Parent or Guardian)

- -

I hereby authorize the Oakland Public Schools to give any and all information contained in the record of:

_____
Name   Birth date

to: Hospital _____
                                        Medical Record Number

Physician _____

Address _____ Telephone _____

_____
(Signature of Parent or Guardian)

13-0125-06   10M171-2

Fig. 5-5. Authorization for Information.

Parent permission for release of information

Medical information is a most important tool for the school nurse, and written permission to obtain this information is protection for the school and nurse from legal proceedings. Parents have the right to make the decision regarding information they are willing to impart to the school. It is usually easier to have these forms signed at the time of registration or during a parent interview (Fig. 5-5).

PROCEDURES AND THE PROCEDURE MANUAL

Procedures must be written so that all school personnel will know exactly what the nurse is doing and why. As a means of critical appraisal of the school nursing program, it is well to carefully think through these activities and to thoroughly understand their value to the schoolchild. For example, a school in a high-income community might not need emphasis on nurse follow-up or a procedure on immunizations or physical and dental examinations for the total school population if the majority of pupils have their own pediatrician and dentist and regularly keep their routine follow-up appointments. The nurse might decide time should be spent on safety education or setting a procedure for working more closely with the teacher, the psychologist, and the parent on mental health or learning disability problems. This specific nursing input is all to the good of pupils, parents, and the school.

Procedures may dictate specific guidelines for health appraisal and follow-up, for vision and hearing conservation, and may extend into the role of the nurse in special education of the handicapped child. All procedures should include the following:

1. *Rationale* for performing procedure
2. *What* is to be done
3. *Who* will be involved
4. *Why*—related to rationale
5. *How* to do procedure
6. *Method* of reporting to others such as the school administrator, school clerk, parent, teacher, physician, guidance counselor, or others intimately involved with the child
7. *Evaluation*—to determine if the procedure is worth the time and effort of school staff for results acquired

Temperature taking is an elementary procedure for nurses; however, in the school setting many other people may take temperatures besides the professional school nurse. In practice, then, it is a good idea to have a procedure that will explain how to use and care for a thermometer. The boxed material describing how to take a temperature and how to care for a thermometer on (p. 46) is such a procedure and is based on the following five points: what to do, why it is done, how to do the procedure, when and to whom to report, and how to evaluate the procedure.

What to do—Use a thermometer to take the child's temperature orally, and then clean and store the thermometer.

Why it is done—This measure protects and isolates an ill child and may prevent spread of disease to other children.

How to do the procedure—The procedure is written to tell how to place the ther-

TEACHER-NURSE CLASSROOM SURVEY

Teacher_____ Grade____ Date_____ Teacher-Nurse Conference
Schedule for_____

Please list below the names of pupils with known or suspected health problems. These
will be discussed at the time of the teacher-nurse conference.

Conditions to note include:

1. Wears Glasses (difficulty seeing,   9. Under Crippled Children Services
    squints, etc.)   10. Allergy (Asthma, Hay Fever)
2. Difficulty Hearing   11. Extreme Nervousness
3. Speech Difficulty   *   12. Known Disease such as Diabetes,
4. On Limited P.E.   Epilepsy, etc.
5. Hearing Condition   13. Nutritional Status - nonbreakfast
6. Dental Problems   eaters
7. Fatigue, listlessness   14. Personal Hygiene
8. Under D.I.G.   15. Attendance Problems

Name	Remarks Concerning Problems	Needs				Under Care
		DT	S	P	M	

Fig. 5-6. Teacher-Nurse Classroom Survey.

mometer for taking temperatures. Caution must be given not to leave small children alone with the thermometer in the mouth. Thermometer must then be cleaned for future use.

When and to whom to report—If temperature is 99.6° F. or over (or what is determined detrimental to the child in school), with or without symptoms, exclude the child. Report to teacher and those responsible for him at school; refer to parent or medical adviser.

How to evaluate procedure—Record results for future tabulation and statistical analysis.

The procedure manual

All procedures and various forms for referral and reporting to parents should be kept in a procedure manual, as well as a sample copy of the Nurses' Daily Report form and other sample forms that pertain to school nursing services. In addition

---

Temperature taking—care of thermometers

Temperatures of students will be taken at the discretion of the school nurse when it is helpful in ascertaining the condition of the student. If temperature is 99.6° F. or over, with or without symptoms, exclude and refer to parent and family medical adviser.

I. Taking temperature
   A. Temperatures are only taken orally.
   B. Rinse thermometers in cold water.
   C. Thermometers should be placed under the tongue with lips closed for three to five minutes. *Small children should not be left alone with thermometer in mouth.*

II. Cleansing and storing thermometers
   A. Rinse thoroughly in cold water.
   B. Wipe down thoroughly with cotton and liquid soap using rotary motion.
   C. Repeat the rinse and place in container of alcohol or benzalkonium chloride (Zephiran).
   D. Thermometers may be stored wet or dry.

III. Reporting a high temperature
   A. Notify parent or person listed on emergency card to come for child or see that the child is transported home.
   B. Notify teacher and principal's office of exclusion.
   C. Confer with person responsible for child about what to do (that is, bed rest, fluids, and calling physician if pupil does not respond to treatment).
   D. Describe conditions in which child can return to school.
   E. Call nurse if further information, advice, medical referral, or other assistance is needed.

IV. Evaluating exclusions
   A. Record number of pupils excluded.
   B. Record results of exclusion.
   C. Describe impact upon other pupils.

to procedures dealing with direct child care, the manual might include the job descriptions and general role and function material on school health personnel. It might also include directions for and information on health instruction and teacher evaluation of pupils (Fig. 5-6).

Periodic review of policies and procedures must be done at least every two years. In some school districts there is a procedure committee composed of representatives of various disciplines and the nurse who meets regularly and makes revisions, additions, and deletions on a continuing basis. A procedure book should be easily available at every school site health office *and kept up-to-date.*

PROCEDURES FOR HEALTH APPRAISAL

Procedures and reports within this chapter were adapted primarily from those developed by the Nursing Services of the Oakland Public Schools; however, material has been included from school districts from all parts of the United States. Although these procedures may seem repetitious, too detailed, or may not exactly fit the needs or programs of a particular school district, adaptations can easily be made.

Procedures for health appraisal include the following: preschool enrollment; medical and dental examinations; health inventories; vision program; color vision screening; machine vision tester; the modified clinical technique (M.C.T.); procedure to expedite program of volunteers for vision screening; hearing program; and vision and hearing conservation. The last procedure combines instructions for both vision and hearing testing and is included to show how the procedures can work together in a unified program.

Preschool enrollment—medical and dental examinations

Preschool enrollment is an ideal time for nurses, volunteers, and school personnel to stress the importance of health in relation to school adjustment and progress, to interpret the school health program to parents, and to encourage periodic medical and dental examinations for all children, not just those who have signs of deformity or illness.

The school department cooperates with parent groups, the medical association, and the county dental society in recommending and securing medical and dental examinations for all kindergarten and new first grade entrants. The school nurse works closely with the parent groups and the school principal in planning the preschool enrollment program.

I. Procedure

A. During the latter part of each school term, certain days are designated for the purpose of preschool enrollment. Each elementary school principal, parent group president, and school nurse receives notification of the dates and instructions regarding the procedure. The parent group president and health chairman and their assistants assist in enrolling the pupils and interviewing their parents.

B. Prior to the enrollment period, the principal may call a group conference or individual conferences with the parent group representatives and the

HEALTH EXAMINATION REPORT OF SCHOOL CHILD

Date _____

Pupil _____ Birth date _____

School _____ Grade _____ Room _____

Dear Parent:

In order that the school can make the best plans for your child's school program, we recommend that you consult your family health adviser and request him to fill out this form and return it to the school.

TO THE DOCTOR:

WE ARE REFERRING THIS PUPIL TO YOU BECAUSE:

☐ Preschool examination ☐ Check-up examination

☐ We are referring this pupil to you because of the following observation:

Referred by _____
NAME   TITLE

PHYSICIAN'S SUMMARY FOR THE SCHOOL

IMMUNIZATIONS AND TESTS (please keep immunizations up-to-date. State date when last given.)

Measles (Rubeola) _____ Had Measles _____
                    Year   Year

Polio initial series _____ Booster _____
                    Number - Year   Month and Year

DPT (diphtheria, pertussis, and tetanus) Series _____ Booster _____
                                          Year   Month and Year

Tetanus _____

Smallpox vaccination (latest) _____

Mumps _____ Had Disease _____
       Year   Year

German Measles (3 day - Rubella) _____ Had Disease _____
                                  Year   Year

Date of last tuberculin skin test _____ Positive _____ Negative(OK) _____

Has he/she had a chest x-ray? _____ BCG vaccine? _____
                              Month and Year   Year

Urinalysis _____ Hemoglobin or Hematocrit _____ Other _____

PERTINENT HEALTH HISTORY, FINDINGS AND RECOMMENDATIONS:

IS THIS PUPIL CURRENTLY UNDER YOUR CARE? ☐ YES ☐ NO

RECOMMENDATIONS FOR PHYSICAL ACTIVITY - ☐ Unrestricted

☐ Restricted activity (please explain) until _____

SPECIAL EDUCATION SERVICES ARE AVAILABLE TO PUPILS WITH HANDICAPPING CONDITIONS. For further information, call the Department of Special Education, 836-2622.

Date of Examination _____

Physician's signature _____

Print name and address _____

DOCTOR: PLEASE FOLD AND RETURN THIS FORM TO SCHOOL AS ADDRESSED ON BACK.

13-0146-10 40M472-1

Fig. 5-7. Health Examination Report of School Child.

A

Name of child_____Birth date_____

School_____Grade_____Room_____

DENTAL EXAMINATION REPORT

	YES	NO	
X-RAY EXAMINATION	☐	☐	Remarks:
PROPHYLAXIS	☐	☐	Remarks:
Topical Fluoride	☐	☐	Remarks:

No dental treatment is necessary at this time ☐ Remarks:

Treatment Plan:

Remarks:

Number of visits anticipated _____ Date of next visit _____

_____ D. D. S.

_____   _____
Date   Address

Doctor: Please fold and return this form to school as addressed on back.

13-0102-06 15M 312-1

B

DENTAL NOTE

_____ School

_____ 19____

To the Parent or Guardian of _____ _____
(Student's Name)   (Grade)

   Your child appears to be in need of dental care. We recommend that you give this matter your attention by making an appointment with your dentist.

_____ P.H.N.
(School Nurse)

   If for any reason you are unable to obtain dental treatment, please consult the school nurse.

13-0128-05 8M1270-8

Fig. 5-8. Dental reports. **A,** Dental Examination Report. **B,** Dental Note.

DISEASE PROTECTION REMINDER

Dear Parent:

According to your child's school health record he/she is unprotected against:

☐ Diphtheria, Whooping Cough, Tetanus (DPT)   ☐ Smallpox   ☐ Polio   ☐ Measles (Rubeola)

☐ Mumps   ☐ German Measles (Rubella)   ☐ Other (specify)

1. Polio—REQUIRED FOR SCHOOL ENROLLMENT BY STATE LAW.
   Polio immunization is recommended for all children during the first year of life and is NOW REQUIRED BEFORE ENTRANCE TO CALIFORNIA SCHOOLS.

2. Measles—REQUIRED FOR SCHOOL ENROLLMENT BY STATE LAW.
   Immunization with attenuated measles vaccine is recommended for any child over nine months of age who have never had measles (Rubeola), and is required before entrance to California schools.

Please fill out form below and return to school. Thank you.

DATE _____   _____, P.H.N.
                                                                      School Nurse

OAKLAND PUBLIC SCHOOLS
Division of Special Services
Department of Health Services

STUDENT'S NAME _____ SCHOOL _____

STUDENT'S TEACHER _____ DATE _____

Please have the student's immunizations brought up-to-date and report the year of the last one for each type or year had disease.

IMMUNIZATION FOR:

Smallpox:
                                    _____   _____
                                    Initial Vaccination   (Date of most recent revaccination)

Diphtheria ⎫
Tetanus   ⎬   _____   _____
Whooping Cough ⎭   Initial Series   (Date of most recent booster)

                                    Please check type   Indicate number   Dates immuniza-
                                    of vaccine   of doses   tions received

Polio:
(Required by law)   _____Oral Monovalent_____   _____

                                    _____Oral Trivalent_____   _____

                                    _____By Injections_____   _____

Measles (Rubeola)   _____ or _____
                                    Date of Immunization   Date Had Disease

Mumps   _____ or _____
                                    Date of Immunization   Date Had Disease

German Measles (Rubella)   _____ or _____
                                    Date of Immunization   Date Had Disease

Other (specify)   _____   _____
                                    Immunization   Date

                                    _____
                                    Signature of Parent or Doctor
13-0170-8 10M771-2   _____

Fig. 5-9. Disease Protection Reminder.

school personnel—nurse and secretary—who will participate. This conference may be used as a means of the following:

1. Assigning each member of the group a definite responsibility
2. Assisting workers in interpreting to parents the value of preschool examinations—pointing out how information obtained may assist parent and school
3. Emphasizing the importance of obtaining *complete* medical information on the Pupil Identification sheet of the Cumulative Record—immunizations, communicable diseases, and other health history
4. Interpreting immunization data (DPT, etc.)

C. Preschool enrollment
1. It is suggested that the school nurse arrange a display of pertinent health literature from which parents may select topics of interest to them.
2. The following forms are given to parents at time of enrollment:
   a. Health Examination Report of School Child (Fig. 5-7)
   b. Dental Report (Fig. 5-8)
   c. Disease Protection Reminder (Fig. 5-9)
3. A Pre-enrollment Report is kept by the school secretary until the end of the registration period (one month) of the following term and then is given to school nurse.

II. Follow-up

A. Medical and dental examination reports are sent to nurse as returned.
B. Appropriate follow-up is done on any defects noted, including referrals, interpretation, and arrangements for school adjustment.

III. Recording

A. Medical and dental examination reports are filed in the pupil's Cumulative Record Folder. Record any defects or state if examination is negative under column "Medical Findings and Recommendations."
B. Nurse records immunization and health history given on Pupil Identification sheet on health record. When there is a discrepancy between immunization dates on Pupil Identification sheet and Health Examination Report of School Child, the dates of the latter will be recorded.
C. Six weeks after the opening of the school term, the nurse should give the kindergarten teachers a list of the names of the children whose medical and dental forms have not been returned. The teacher will be instructed to send a "reminder" letter to parents along with the appropriate forms.

IV. Term report

A. A report of preschool examinations is made to the principal and the school health services at the end of the semester. This report includes the following:
1. Total number of new kindergarten enrollments
2. Number of Health Examination Report of School Child forms returned
3. Number of Dental Report forms of preschool children returned

HEALTH INVENTORY FOR ELEMENTARY PUPILS

Name_____ Grade_____ Teacher_____ School_____

To Parents: Please fill out and return this form tomorrow. This information is used in the school program to promote and protect the health of students.

I. Immunization History: Give month and year completing immunizations for:

Measles vaccination (Rubeola)_____ Had Disease_____
                                                YEAR   YEAR

Polio initial series_____ Booster_____
                              NUMBER – YEAR   MONTH AND YEAR

DPT (diphtheria, pertussis and tetanus) Series_____ Booster_____
                                                  YEAR   MONTH AND YEAR

Tetanus (Latest)_____
                                                      YEAR

Smallpox vaccination (Latest)_____
                                                          YEAR

A

Mumps vaccination_____ Had Disease_____
                                    YEAR   YEAR

German Measles (3 day-Rubella)_____ Had Disease_____
                                          YEAR   YEAR

Date of last tuberculin skin test_____Positive_____Negative (OK)_____

Has he/she had a chest x-ray?_____ BCG vaccine?_____
                              MONTH AND YEAR   YEAR

II. History of Illness: Give age

____ Anemia	____ Diabetes	____ Heart Disease	____ Rheumatic fever
____ Asthma	____ German Measles	____ Hernia (Rupture)	____ Skin Problems
____ Chicken Pox	____ Hay fever	____ Measles	____ Tuberculosis
____ Convulsions	____ Hearing Problem	____ Mumps	____ Vision Problem

Surgery_____ Injury_____

Any other serious illness?_____

PLEASE COMPLETE OTHER SIDE
(Front)

Fig. 5-10. **A** and **B,** Health Inventory for Elementary Pupils. **C** and **D,** Health Inventory for Secondary School Students.

III. History of Symptoms: Give age

___ Frequent colds or   ___ Frequent use of toilet   ___ Angers easily
___ sore throats   ___ Frequent stomach ache   ___ Worries a great deal
___ Nosebleeds   ___ Toothaches   ___ Many fears
___ Persistent cough   ___ Frequent pains in legs   ___ Nervousness
___ Running ear   ___ Bedwetting   ___ Tires easily
___ Frequent headache

IV. Medical and Dental Care:

Name of child's doctor or clinic _____

MEDICAL RECORD NO.

_____
ADDRESS

Date of most recent visit _____ Reason for visit _____

_____

Name of child's dentist or dental clinic _____

_____
ADDRESS

B Date of last visit _____

Was all necessary dental work completed?   _____   _____
                                              YES   NO

V. Are there any other health problems or family matters which you think would be helpful for the school to know? _____

_____

_____

_____

_____

_____

_____
PARENT-S SIGNATURE

_____   _____
DATE   HOME TELEPHONE

13-0150-09 20M771-3

(Back)

Continued.

Fig. 5-10, cont'd. For legend see opposite page.

HEALTH INVENTORY FOR SECONDARY SCHOOL STUDENTS

Name_____ Birth date_____Phone_____

School_____Counselor_____Grade_____Home Room_____

TO THE STUDENT:

It is important that you become familiar with reporting your health history. Health records are significant in planning school programs. Please fill out and return this form. Consult with your parents for the answers, if necessary.

1. Please give name of your physician or medical clinic_____

2. For what reason and when were you last examined?_____

3. Are you now taking medication?_____What are you taking?_____Why?_____

4. Do you wear glasses?_____Date of last examination by eye doctor_____

5. Have you ever had a serious illness, accident, or operation? Please describe and tell when_____
_____

6. State any reason you should not take regular physical education_____
_____

C

7. Do you think you are in good health?_____

8. Please check any of the following which trouble you:

____Headaches	____Poor vision	____Poor hearing	____German measles
____More than 4 colds a year	____Toothaches	____Hay fever	____Measles
____Pains in legs or joints	____Persistent cough	____Acne (pimples)	____Mumps
____Tired during the day	____Shortness of breath	____Cavities in teeth	____Chicken pox
____Asthma	____Epilepsy	____Diabetes	____Scarlet fever

Is there anything else which troubles you?_____

9. Have you had a urine test?_____Was it normal?_____

10. Have you had a blood test?_____Was it normal?_____

11. Year of last vaccination for smallpox_____

12. Year of last immunization for diphtheria and tetanus_____

13. Year of last immunization for polio_____How many oral doses?_____How many shots?_____

14. Year of immunization for measles_____Other immunizations (specify)_____
_____

PLEASE COMPLETE OTHER SIDE

13-0172-05 10M1171-2

(Front)

Fig. 5-10, cont'd. For legend see p. 52.

15. Have you ever been exposed to anyone with tuberculosis?_____Year_____

Have you had a skin test for tuberculosis?_____Year_____Results: Positive____Negative____

Have you ever had a chest x-ray?_____Year_____What was the report?_____

16. Name of dentist_____Date of last visit_____Do you need dental

care at present?_____

17. What time do you usually go to bed?_____Do you usually get as much sleep as you like?_____

If not, what usually keeps you from getting it?_____

_____

18. Do you eat breakfast?_____Always_____Part of the time_____Seldom_____

19. Do you have a job?_____

20. Do you discuss your health problems with your parents? Always_____, part of the time_____seldom_____

21. At the present time, do you have any questions or problems which you would like to discuss with nurse_____,

vice principal_____, your counselor_____guidance consultant_____.

22. Check any of the following items about which you are concerned and for which you would like help: Awkwardness_____,

too big physically_____, underdeveloped_____, having to dress for gym_____, social problems_____, unable to sleep

D   at night_____. List any other problems or concerns_____

_____

_____

_____   _____
Student's signature   DATE

(Back)

Fig. 5-10, cont'd. For legend see p. 52.

Health inventories

The need for health information about each student is essential to assist him in making his best adjustment to school. This information also assists the school staff in program planning and health supervision in the school.

I. **General recommendations**

    A. Individual schools should establish a routine procedure within the framework of the department of health services to obtain health information.

    B. A Health Inventory form should be secured on each student in preschool or grades kindergarten or first, seventh, tenth, or as needed (Fig. 5-10, *A* and *B*).

    C. All students should be urged to obtain a medical report from their physicians or clinic at entrance to school and entrance to junior and senior high school.

II. **Procedure**

    A. Elementary school nurse, in cooperation with the school administrator and the Parent-Teacher Association or other volunteer groups, obtains preschool medical and dental reports for all kindergarten (or first grade) pupils. Preschool reports are acceptable.

    B. The nurse should request the secondary student to fill out a Health Inventory form or ask the parent to complete it for elementary pupils.

    C. Routine requests for medical examinations of graduating sixth and ninth grade students are encouraged, but this is optional according to the circumstances at the individual school. Health Examination Report of School Child and Dental Report forms are shown in Figs. 5-7 and 5-8.

    D. Pertinent information is made immediately available to school personnel. A periodic report, at least annually, of the particular physical problem that qualifies a student for special education will be recorded by the nurse.

    E. Health information reports are placed in the Cumulative Folder. Only pertinent information will be transcribed to the permanent health record.

Vision program

The purpose of a vision screening program is to discover and ensure proper correction of eye defects as early as possible and to make appropriate adjustments in the student's school program as well as to provide positive learning experiences in eye health for all students. Several vision screening procedures are described here. Selection of the appropriate procedure is the decision of the school district.

I. **Vision screening procedure**

    A. Selection of pupils

        1. All students in grades kindergarten and thereafter as prescribed by law or the school district

2. All pupils new to the school district, without a vision test
3. Pupils referred due to signs and symptoms of visual difficulty
4. Pupils being referred to special services for any reason, who have not had a vision test within the last year

B. Nursing responsibilities
1. Vision screening is the responsibility of the nurse in the school, and appropriate arrangements should be made with teachers and administrators to facilitate the program.
2. Ideally, the tests are given upon completion of the unit of health instruction dealing with the eye. Audiovisual aids should be available.

C. Testing of pupils
1. Snellen test
   a. Use Good-Lite Snellen E chart with cover card in elementary schools. In secondary schools, alphabet or E charts may be used.
   b. Each eye is tested separately.
   c. Visual acuity 20/40 or less in one or both eyes should be rechecked and referred to eye specialist.
   d. It is permissible for one letter to be missed on line 20/20 and one letter on preceding lines.
   e. Note symptoms of strabismus, tilting of head, etc., recheck, and refer to eye specialist.
2. Color vision testing
   a. Test once in elementary grades.
   b. Use pseudoisochromatic plates available and follow directions from source of purchase.
   c. Use score sheet only on those pupils who fail color test.

II. Follow-up

A. The school nurse will confer with parents, either at school or in the home, on defects discovered and assist in arranging satisfactory facilities for care.
1. Families should be referred to their usual source of eye care on the Eye Examination Referral form (Fig. 5-11).
2. Families needing financial assistance should be referred to part-pay or free resources in the community. These resources change and eligibility varies each year, so maintain current file for latest information.

B. Parents should be informed that plastic and shatterproof lenses are available wherever glasses are obtained.

C. All referrals for examinations should be made on Eye Examination Referral form. For severe defects, see procedure on special services for partially sighted or blind, p. 89.

D. Keep teachers, counselor, and administrator informed of the results of the vision tests, follow-up action, and eye examiner's recommendation. Recording on the Cumulative Health Record form (Fig. 5-1) is not usually done until follow-up is completed.

Text continued on p. 62.

Date_____

School_____

Address_____

REFERRAL FOR EYE EXAMINATION

DEAR PARENT:

A recent vision test at school indicates that_____
(name of pupil)

may have some vision difficulty. An eye examination is urgently recommended. Kindly take this form with you at the time of the examination.

_____
Nurse

TO THE EYE EXAMINER:

We are referring this pupil to you for the following reason:

Failed the Snellen Test_____ R. 20/   L. 20/

Signs and symptoms of visual problems_____

EYE EXAMINER'S REPORT TO THE SCHOOL

A

I.   Visual acuity (a) without correction R. 20/   L. 20/

(b) with correction   R. 20/   L. 20/

(c) Jaeger reading (near vision acuity)

II.   Glasses: ☐ Prescribed   ☐ Not prescribed   Unbreakable: Yes___ No___

☐ To be worn all of the time   To be used in games & sports: Yes___ No___

☐ To be worn for close work only   ☐ To be worn for distance only

III.   Diagnosis and/or etiology _____

IV.   When should the student return for a re-examination?_____

V.   Comments_____

_____

_____

VI.   If this pupil needs special education under the program for the partially sighted, a more detailed report is required (see reverse side regarding standards for this program). Please check below if you recommend this service and the required form will be forwarded to you for completion.

_____Recommend program for the partially sighted.

Date_____   _____
Eye Examiner

_____
Address or clinic

Note to Examiner: Please mail completed form to school indicated above.

13-0147-05 15M465-1

(Front)

Fig. 5-11. Eye Examination Referral.

STANDARDS FOR ASSIGNMENT TO PROGRAM OF INSTRUCTION FOR PARTIALLY SEEING CHILDREN

1. Visual acuity of 20/70 or less in the better eye with correction.

2. Following eye surgery in cases in which re-adaptation of eye use is necessary.

3. Muscle anomalies, especially strabismus, in cases in which re-education of the deviating eye is necessary.

4. Other visual deviations which, in the opinion of the eye specialist, can benefit from special education facilities.

B

(Back)

Fig. 5-11, cont'd. For legend see opposite page.

Nurse_____   Date_____

VISION TESTING

GRADE	TEACHER	SNELLEN				PLUS SPHERE				SIGNS AND SYMPTOMS		
		NUMBER TESTED	FAILED*	GLASSES OBTAINED	GLASSES NOT NECESSARY	NUMBER TESTED	FAILED**	GLASSES OBTAINED	GLASSES NOT NECESSARY	NUMBER	GLASSES OBTAINED	GLASSES NOT NECESSARY

A

*Sees 20/40 or less (Snellen) in both or either eye
**Sees 20/20 line (Plus Sphere) in both or either eye
Signs and Symptoms but passing Snellen and Plus Sphere

THIS SAME FORM IS TO BE USED FOR THE TERM REPORT

13-0152-01 14M155-1

Fig. 5-12. Vision Testing.

VISION TESTING

Teacher _____ Grade _____ Enrollment _____ Date _____

	Snellen Test Without Glasses R L	Snellen Test With Glasses R L	Color Test	Signs and Symptom	Referral see below	Follow-up (see below)	Remarks (Reason for lack of follow-up, etc.)
1.	Retest						
2.	Retest						
3.	Retest						
4.	Retest						
5.	Retest						
6.	Retest						
7.	Retest						
8.	Retest						
9.	Retest						
10.	Retest						

B

Directions
Referral: O – Old case – previously referred & under care
N – Previously referred but not yet under care
R – Referred to eye specialist & Defect Card made out (new case)

Follow-up: E – Examined & glasses not needed
G – Examined & glasses obtained
N – Has not obtained care

Absentees: No findings after name indicates absent for test

Fig. 5-12, cont'd. For legend see opposite page.

III. Records and reports

A. Results of tests are usually first recorded on the Vision Testing Roster (Fig. 5-12).
   1. Snellen: R 20/20 L 20/20
   2. Color vision: passed ___; failed ___. Add score sheet to Cumulative Health Record for those pupils who fail color test.
   3. Nurses' Follow-Up Record cards are made on all pupils failing tests or with unusual signs and symptoms of eye defects (Fig. 5-2, *A* and *B*).
   4. Include information on follow-up card needed for the annual report to facilitate completion at the end of the school year. Data should include:
      a. Where and when under care (if already seen by eye specialist)
      b. Where and when referred for care
      c. Results of referral (glasses, recommendations of eye specialist, reasons for no follow-up by families)

Color vision screening

Color vision defects may affect school progress and vocational choice. Since the defect is so rare among girls, only boys are routinely tested. It is desirable to test all males once during elementary grades. For district-wide continuity it is recommended that all boys in kindergarten or first grade be tested. This test does not need to be repeated.

I. Preliminary procedures

A. Using cards with three symbols, $\times$ $\bigcirc$ $\triangle$, in black on white, teacher holds up individual symbols and each student practices finding respective symbols on his card.
B. Put the large card on the table in this fashion: $\boxed{\times \bigcirc \triangle}$
C. Now hold up the folded card so that one object at a time may be seen.
D. Ask boy to find the matching figure on the large card in the following manner:

$\boxed{\triangle}$

Teacher holds this up.

$\boxed{\times \bigcirc \triangle}$

Child points to symbol.

II. Equipment

A. American Optical Corp. H. R. R. plates.
B. American Optical Corp. blue-filtered light or daylight fluorescent tube in desk lamp.
C. Almost dark room, no artificial lighting (Testing should be done in a secluded area.)

III. Testing procedure

Child should use his own three-symbol card to identify symbols seen on plates. The book should be tilted up in a position similar to reading position on table with the prescribed light on the plate and the child standing immediately in front of book approximately 30 inches from book. The screener should encourage child by saying, "What can you find on this page?"

A. Preliminary evaluation: demonstration screening plates A B C D (to ascertain if child understands test). Be sure to advise child that plate D has nothing on it.

B. Routine screening
   1. Basic plates 1 through 6 (exclude plate 3 with kindergarten and first graders)
   2. Mild red-green defect, plates 7 through 11
   3. Medium red-green defect, plates 12 through 14
   4. Strong red-green defect, plates 15 and 16
   5. Blue-yellow defect, plates 17 through 20

C. For less lengthy procedure, if the student misses even one symbol on plates 4, 5, or 6, the screener may turn immediately to plates 15 and 16 (strong defect plates), and if student passes 15 and 16, then screener may proceed through plates 7 through 11 (mild red-green defect) and plates 12 through 14 (medium red-green defect).

IV. Testing results

A. Normal: correctly identifies plates 1 through 6

B. Mild red-green defect: incorrectly identifies some items on plates 7 through 11, but passes 12 through 16

C. Medium red-green defect: incorrectly identifies some items on plates 12 through 14, but passes 15 and 16

D. Strong red-green defect: incorrectly identifies some items on plates 15 and 16

E. Blue-yellow defect: incorrectly identifies some items on plates 17 through 20 (very rare)

NOTE: Defect in color vision may be based on missing only one symbol on any plate.

V. Follow-up

A. Type of color defect

B. Record on child's health card
   1. Color vision: normal
   2. Color vision: mild, medium, strong red-green or blue-yellow defect

C. Initiate defect cards on all suspected failures

D. Child's family should be informed of possible defect by conference, telephone, or note and implications regarding vocational choices.

E. Teachers should be informed of test results and reminded each subsequent year.

F. It should be stressed that there is no treatment for color vision defect.

Machine Vision Tester

The Vision Tester is a precision built optical instrument designed for rapid and precise measurement of visual performance. Types of testing done with the machines are right and left acuity, vertical and lateral imbalance, and color blindness. You may purchase other slides, but the slides mentioned are sufficient for good screening.

Standards for referral vary. In areas where professional services are readily available, the preference often is for a standard such as 20/20 or above in each eye, while below 20/20 in either eye is a referral. Basically it is recommended that standards for referral be established on local ophthalmic professional advice. In areas where relatively few children have had eye care and where professional services are not as readily available, 20/30 in each eye seems to be the standard accepted as normal or not in need of immediate attention.

Correlation between sight and subjects taught in school is endless, and constant correlation should be made. Health, safety, art, language arts, and many others can be used for teaching purposes in the school.

Grade: 1 through 12 (primary and secondary)
Topic: Use of Machine Vision Tester
Concept: To obtain as near as possible accurate vision screening results for swift and proper referrals for the conservation of sight.

I. Description of activity

The young child ready for his first vision screening must be well prepared in advance by exposing him to the "E" charts and by being very imaginative in teaching the directional "E." You may call the "E" a table with three legs or show them how to arrange the three middle fingers to form an "E." When and only when the directional "E" is thoroughly understood are you ready to start testing.

II. Skillful testing

A. Familiarize yourself with the instrument and with each test before you start testing.
 1. Look through the instrument and learn for yourself what happens when the occluder switches are turned and when the lens lever is moved from far to near.
 2. Get the habit of resetting the dial, lens lever, and occluding switches for test I as soon as you finish testing a pupil.
B. Make the pupil feel comfortable and at ease.
 1. Learn the habit of adjusting the instrument quickly and easily for different heights of pupils.
 2. See that the pupil's chair is close enough to the table so that he is comfortable. It may help to have him place his arms on the table. (It is often desirable to have the student stand, since it saves a good deal of time.)
 3. Face the subject while testing. It will induce better response.
C. Handling the subject.
 1. Greet each pupil pleasantly.

2. State questions clearly, slowly, and firmly.
3. Encourage each child to do his best, by voice and manner.
4. Do not say "that is right" or "that is wrong" when he answers your questions. He may confuse "right" with "left"—or with the direction in which the "E" points.

D. Keep each pupil's attention on the tests.
1. Do not let the pupil continue looking at a test slide after the test has been finished. Proceed immediately.
2. Skill in eliciting correct responses from young children is an art that varies with individuals. The tester should feel free to vary the test questions with first grade or preschool children to put the child at ease and to stimulate his desire to respond. In testing children in the third grade and above, the tester can be more direct with questions and get positive answers.
3. When a child hesitates or indicates that he does not see clearly, ask him to guess the direction in which the fingers of the "E" point. Often this is the only way to obtain a clear demonstration of ability or inability to read a given line.
4. Pointing to a specific test symbol is vital. Do not let the pointer move aimlessly around it.

The modified clinical technique

The importance of a procedure such as the modified clinical technique (M.C.T.) can be seen in the Orinda study done by Hendrix Blum in 1959. The M.C.T. is a case-finding procedure that identifies virtually all the vision problems that might interfere with school progress. The battery of tests include distance vision (Snellen), binocular coordination, refractive error (focus), color vision, and possible eye disease. Failure means a referral for a complete vision examination by an eye practitioner. These referrals and follow-up are made by the school nurse. The results of this study have been slowly assimilated into the operation of schools, mostly in California.

The M.C.T. is usually given to kindergarten children or whenever the child first enters school. The procedure for testing has been carefully planned and the program usually runs smoothly on testing days with the assistance of two or three volunteers. The M.C.T. is scheduled in advance and is performed by an optometrist who is assigned to the school. There is a fee for testing services, dependent on the time necessary to do the testing. Most school districts utilizing this service are satisfied with its results. The only barriers seem to be cost and that some ophthalmologists feel there are too many referrals, although there is no reliable data to prove this.

Procedure to expedite program of volunteers for vision screening

The Vision Screening Request form is submitted to health services by the school nurse upon receiving approval for same from principal.

I. Assignment of volunteers

A team of volunteers is then assigned to the school. The team is composed of women who have received instruction from a consultant from the Society for Prevention of Blindness in simple vision testing and have had a supervised practice session. The nurse will be informed of the initial scheduled date of visitation by the volunteer team.

II. Responsibilities of the school nurse

A. Keep principal informed of dates of visitation by volunteer team to screen and/or retest.
B. Schedule classes to be screened and inform teachers regarding program.
   1. Have teachers prepare an identification card for each student, including full name and birth date (rather than age), and pin on student at time of screening.
   2. Remind teachers to send School Health Records in care of an adult at the time of screening to the screening area (not to be carried by individual student). Recording will be done by volunteers.
   3. Urge teachers to teach "E" game prior to screening date wherever feasible.
C. Select suitable area for screening to be done. Provide Snellen eye chart and cover cards.
D. Make arrangements with volunteer team for return dates to complete screening and/or retests. Nurses who have an additional school or schools may want to set dates with the team for testing at these sites. Such dates will have to be on an individual basis, since they must be mutually agreeable.
E. Send following educational material home with students in classrooms when screening has been completed.
   1. Letter for parent
   2. Leaflet, "Signs of Eye Trouble"
F. Follow-up of discovered or suspected vision problems will be by usual procedure with exceptions as listed below. Give to parent:
   1. Eye Referral form in triplicate (NOTE: This form is supplied by the Society for Prevention of Blindness. Use this referral form *only* when referring students tested under the volunteer program. Students not tested by volunteers for vision screening but needing follow-up should be referred on the usual school referral forms.) Nurse will keep one report for Cumulative Folder. Send duplicates to health services.
   2. Self-addressed envelope for return of above by examining eye doctor.
   3. Release of Information form supplied by the Society for Prevention of Blindness.
   4. Pamphlet, "Charlie Brown, Detective."
G. Report to be sent to the Society for Prevention of Blindness.
   1. *Keep all master sheets* (when completed by volunteer team after each screening session) *at school site at all times.* (Reports to the Society for Prevention of Blindness will be drawn from these forms.)

Hearing program

The purpose of the hearing conservation program is to detect the student with a hearing loss as soon as possible in order to advise the family regarding adequate follow-up procedures to correct and compensate for this loss and to make appropriate adjustments in the student's school program.

I. **Hearing screening procedure**

A. Audiometric testing is done by the school audiometrists or the trained school nurse or assistant. They prepare the schedule for testing at the schools each semester.
1. All students are tested in selected grades as determined by the school district.
2. Pupils in other grades or special classes, for whom a hearing test is recommended, may also be included at the request of the nurse or teacher.
B. Students who fail the group test receive an individual threshold test at the school within a short time. *Only those students who fail the individual threshold test are reported as having probable hearing losses.*
C. The audiograms of all students who fail the threshold test are sent with a referral for examinations by ear specialists.
D. The otologist examines students and recommends for special educational assignments.

II. **Nursing responsibilities**

A. Check with the principal for testing dates.
B. Compile a list of students with suspected hearing losses in grades not in the

GROUP HEARING TEST REPORT

Name _____

Date of Birth _____ Sex _____ Date _____

School _____ Grade _____ Counselor/or Teacher _____

RIGHT EAR	FREQUENCIES	LEFT EAR
	500	
	1000	
	2000	
	4000	
	6000	
	8000	

Comments: _____

Fig. 5-13. Group Hearing Test Report.

routine testing schedule, and notify tester for audiometrist of the number of these referrals.

C. When the list of failures from the group test is received, individual threshold testing is done on these pupils at the school. For examples of group test and threshold test forms, see Figs. 5-13 and 5-14.

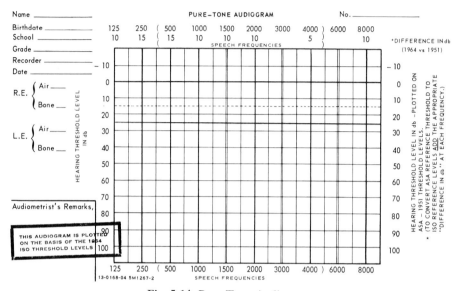

Fig. 5-14. Pure-Tone Audiogram.

HEARING LOSS NOTE AND RECOMMENDATIONS ON SEATING

TO THE TEACHERS:

Students with hearing losses are usually sensitive about it, and the teachers are requested to talk to the student privately, explaining the reason for changing his seat, etc.

Special recommendations for this student are:

Right ear to teacher_____   Left ear to teacher_____

Seat front_____

Student_____ _____ Grade_____ Date_____

Director
Department of Health Services

13-0158-01 15M357-2

Fig. 5-15. Hearing Loss Note and Recommendations on Seating.

D. Upon receipt of an audiogram of a student who shows a loss on the individual threshold test, school nurse follow-up commences by completing a follow-up card if one does not already exist.

E. Refer to appropriate source of care.

F. Copies of audiograms will be sent to the doctor.

REQUEST FOR SPECIAL SERVICE

Date..19.........

NAME.. Birth Date.......................... Sex.......... School..................................
(Last Name)   (First Name)

Address.. Phone No...

Father's Name..Occupation...............................Mother's Name..Occupation..........................

Made out by:..Referred by..
(Principal or Vice-Principal)

TO BE REFERRED TO:

Attendance.................... Health Services.................... Ind. Guidance.....................Occ. Adjustment....................... Special Ed..................... Research..................

REASON FOR REFERRAL (State Problem Specifically).

....
....
....

SCHOOL STATUS

Grade:........................ Date ent. this school........................From (school)...............................No. schools attended..........................

Quality of school work: Poor....................... Average.................... Good................... Best work in:....................... Poorest work in:...................

Prior attendance record: Definitely good..................... Doubtful.................... Definitely bad ....

TEST DATA (Individual and group, intelligence and achievement)

Date	School	Test Form	Score	C.A.	M.A.	A.A.	Ratio

PHYSICAL DEVELOPMENT AND HEALTH OBSERVATION

Short for age.......... Average......... Tall............ Underweight............ Average........... Overweight............ Looks delicate........... Average........... Robust..........

Seldom ill..................... Average amount of illness.................... Frequently ill..................... Recent severe illness..................... Easily fatigued..................

Vision defect.................................. Hearing defect........................... Speech defect...................... ... Dental defect..................

Physical peculiarities........................

SOCIAL-PERSONAL RECORD

Special interests..

Special difficulties..

Friends..

Participation in classroom..

Participation on playground..

Out-of-school interests...

Employment..

Behavior Pattern: (Describe pupil's behavior—use reverse side of sheet for additional information)

....
....
....
....
....

HOME

Attitude of parents toward child:..

Attitude of parents toward school:...

Broken home.................... Stepfather..................... Stepmother...................... Foster home...................

Relatives and others in home:... Language spoken in home:...................

Other children in family:

Name	School	Age	Name	School	Age

A

13-0107-05 10M566-7   **(Front)**

Continued.

Fig. 5-16. Request for Special Service.

COMMENTS:

REPORT FROM NURSE:

    a. Vision test: Type..Date of Test..R................L................

    b. Hearing test: Type..Date of Test..R................L................

    c. Date of physical examination and summary:

B

    d. Other pertinent facts:

....
(Nurse's Signature)

FOR SPECIAL CLASS PLACEMENT ONLY:

    a. Name of teacher to whose class pupil will be assigned..

    b. Present number of pupils in the class..

(Back)

Fig. 5-16, cont'd. For legend see p. 69.

G. Nurse should obtain a follow-up report from the doctor on all students with hearing loss.

H. The classroom teacher should be instructed for preferential seating both verbally and in writing (Fig. 5-15).

I. If special education services are recommended and student is not already receiving them, attach to Request for Special Service form (Fig. 5-16).

III. Recording

A. The school nurse does not record group test results. Group tests "passed" are recorded by classroom teacher.

B. A stamp is available for use immediately after testing is done in the school.

C. Group test "failures" are recorded by the audiometrist.

D. Threshold test results are recorded by the nurse.

E. Summary of medical finding reports are recorded by the nurse on the health section of the Cumulative Folder (refer to Fig. 5-2, *A* and *B*).

Vision and hearing conservation

If a child is to achieve to the best of his ability or to his optimum, he must possess a feeling of *well-being*. Well-being is derived from good physical, social, and emotional health. Impaired hearing or vision will handicap in one or all three of the above areas mentioned, thus preventing the child's functioning in a manner acceptable to himself or to others. The ability to hear or to see properly is directly related to the ability to learn and to gain enjoyment in life.

I. Objectives

A. To identify pupils with certain vision and hearing (or both) difficulties such as may be found by:

VISION	HEARING
1. Snellen eye test	1. Audiometric testing
2. Teacher or nurse observation	2. Teacher or nurse observation
3. Parental statements or requests	3. Parental statements or requests
4. Complaints of the child	4. Complaints of the child

B. To refer, assist, and follow up all vision and hearing defects or deviations from the normal until the child is able to function within normal limits or to capacity under his particular degree of vision and/or hearing handicap:

ACCEPTABLE VISION	ACCEPTABLE HEARING
1. 20/20 to 20/30 Snellen test	1. Loss of less than 20 db in 2 frequencies in one ear
2. No apparent deviation	2. Loss of less than 30 db in any frequencies
	3. No evidence of pathology that might lead to hearing loss

C. Criteria for referral:

VISION	HEARING
1. 20/30 Snellen test	1. Loss of more than 20 db in 2 frequencies in one ear
2. Deviation	
3. Learning difficulties	2. Loss of more than 20 db in any frequency
	3. Evidence of irregular physical or pathological conditions pertaining to the ear

II. Responsibility and techniques

The role of the nurse is to foster, protect, and promote conditions conducive to maintaining and conserving the sight and hearing of individuals under care. Good rapport and a sense of humor aid in relating to everyday associates and contacts in the area of screening, planning (referral), implementing, evaluating, and study and research. She assumes the responsibility for screening of vision and hearing procedures used in health appraisal and the follow-up on all matters pertaining to the health care of the school-age child. The "follow-up" of the screening program is carried out in the three phases.

A. Phase I
   1. Cooperation and coordination of everyone essential to vision and hearing team
   2. Swift referral of vision and/or hearing defects to the proper medical source
   3. Knowledge of the community resources that can assist and meet referral needs
   4. Contact with those qualified to provide special educational needs
B. Phase II: Recognition that a good screening program is not for diagnostic purposes.
C. Phase III: The needs for periodic reevaluation of methods and techniques used in vision and hearing screening programs and the screener be well trained and prepared.

III. Rationale

The early detection of possible defects of vision and hearing is imperative and often has great bearing on the prognosis of future performances; prognosis improves by early referral.

A. Color blindness: Tests should be run in the early school years to aid the teachers and the child in special adjustments.

IV. Priority

Vision and hearing must be adopted into school health and education as a *high-priority* program to ensure all possible protection to the two vital senses (vision and hearing). Proper functioning of these two senses is the foundation for security in any individual's pursuits in life.

A. Priority: Visual or hearing education for advanced loss
1. Tools or equipment
2. Emotional or mental health needs
3. Occupational training priorities
B. Screening priority
1. First priority for screening should go to the 4- to 6-year-old children and/or the first grades.
2. Second priority should go to grades three and four.
If only one grade per year can be screened, the first grade should have priority. If screening of two grades is possible, the third would be a good second priority.

VISION SCREENING

I. Grades kindergarten through twelfth

Subject: Vision testing
Topic: Snellen vision testing
Concept: Our overall objective of the school vision screening program is to identify pupils with vision difficulties early and make proper referral for the conservation of sight.

A. Equipment
1. A Snellen chart, preferably self-illuminating
2. A large symbol "E" mounted on cardboard
3. A window card (not recommended by some eye specialists)
4. An adequate translucent occluding device, such as clean 3 × 5 inch cards
5. Forms for recording results
6. A light meter
B. Arrangement of equipment for testing
Hang the Snellen cabinet or chart at one end of the room where there is at least 21 feet of clear floor space immediately in front of it. Mark on the floor a line 20 feet distant from and directly in front of the chart. The location that pupils will occupy while they are being tested will then be back of this line at a point where their eyes are directly over the line and 20 feet from the chart. The height at which the chart is hung on the wall should be adjusted so that the center is at approximately the pupil's eye level. Some charts are on adjustable stands.
C. Description of the test
The Snellen test is given with a chart that has either a number of letters of the alphabet of specified sizes printed in rows or only the letter "E" of specified sizes and in various positions printed in rows. In each instance the symbol on the top line of the chart is of such size that, under testing conditions, a person with normal vision is able to identify the letter or tell its position from a distance of 200 feet. In each succeeding row from the top row downward, the size of the symbols is reduced to a point that a person with normal vision can see them at a distance of 100, 70, 50, 40, 30, 20, and 15 feet, respectively.
D. Administering the Snellen test
In order to secure the confidence, understanding, and cooperation of pupils

when they are taking the test for the first time, explain to them the purpose and procedures. With very young children who have never taken a vision test, demonstrate the procedure with the large symbol "E"; turn "E" to various positions and, as it is held in each position, show the pupils how to indicate the direction in which the legs of the "E" point. This procedure may be carried on in the spirit of a game: The pupils indicate with both arms the direction in which the "legs" of the "table" are pointing. The pretesting activities may be carried out in regular classrooms.

Pupils who are far enough along in school that they can be relied upon to report verbally the direction in which the symbol points may be taught to respond by saying, "left," "right," "up," or "down." However, they may be permitted to indicate the positions by pointing.

E. Room and environment

The room should be large enough that the Snellen chart can be hung on a wall and have at least 21 feet of clear floor space directly in front of the chart.

The room should be equipped so that the light can be controlled to secure the intensity necessary. It should be located where it is relatively quiet, and it should be free of internal conditions that may be distracting to children being tested. Visual acuity increases as the intensity of light increases, until a level is reached that causes eye discomfort; and visual acuity decreases as the intensity of light decreases. It is therefore important to have the chart used for testing vision properly lighted at all times. Lighted Snellen chart cabinets (self-illuminating charts) that provide 10 footcandles of evenly diffused light on the chart face are recommended for use in the vision screening program.

F. Testing

1. Adopt and employ a standard testing procedure.
2. If the pupil is wearing glasses, it is not necessary to test him routinely.
3. Test the vision in one eye at a time—the right eye first, the left eye next. Use an occluder or hold a small cover card obliquely along the nose of the pupil to cover the eye not being tested. Pupils are to keep both eyes open during the test—the one being tested and the one covered by the card. Care should be taken that the card does not press on the eye.
4. Use a fresh cover card with each pupil so as to prevent any infectious condition from being communicated from one pupil to another.
5. Observe the pupil's eyes as well as the chart. Have an assistant stand beside the chart and frame with a window card the symbol to be read.
6. If no vision difficulty is suspected, have the pupil start reading the "50" line. If the pupil responds readily and correctly to this line, then check his performance on the "20" line.

G. Criteria for referral

Each pupil whose performance on the Snellen test indicates vision difficulty or who, as observed and reported by the teacher or nurse, evidences vision difficulty should be retested and the findings reappraised before the school recommends an eye examination. The retesting and reappraisal should be done by the school nurse or other qualified person within ten days after the results of the first screening test or the teacher's report has been received.

The parents of pupils with 20/40 vision or less in one or both eyes, verified by the retest, should be informed regarding the test results and a recommendation made for them to secure for their child a professional eye examination.

A professional eye examination should be recommended for a pupil who has been found through appropriate and adequate appraisal to have significant signs or symptoms (behavior, appearance, or complaints as indicated previously under "teacher observation") that suggest visual difficulty, even though his performance on the Snellen test is acceptable.

H. Follow-up
1. The problem should be brought to the attention of parents.
2. Contact with parents should be maintained until the pupil has received the needed examination and such care as is necessary.
3. The results of the examination and statement of recommendations from the eye and vision specialist should be made available to the school. The final step is needed by the school as a basis for making any needed adjustments in the pupil's educational program.

II. Vision screening day activity

A. Assign students to each task after giving explanation for the task.
1. Measure 20 feet plus one foot for chair or standing room.
2. Set up chart.
3. Make cover cards, after washing hands with soap.
4. Check light around chart with light meter.
5. Have student find best place in room for chart by checking light and report to other students what he found.
6. Assign one student to call pupils for test, doing it quietly, having them ready on time to avoid any possible delay, and waste of time.
B. Explain that all students may not be able to identify each symbol; if unable to do so, simply say so.
C. Explain that referral for an eye examination does not necessarily mean you need glasses. The doctor will decide.

HEARING AND AUDIOMETERS

I. Objective

To obtain accurate audiograms for detecting hearing losses and making necessary referrals as soon as possible.

II. Materials needed

A. Audiometer and earphones
B. Audio graph chart
C. Quiet room

III. Preparation for testing

Explain to the young child that he will hear five sounds similar to sounds heard by jet pilots and telephone operators, first in the right ear and then in the left ear. These sounds will start loud and then decrease in volume. Show children earphones and how they are placed on the ears. They may indicate whether or not they hear sound either by saying "yes" or "no" or by raising hands. Follow with individual demonstration and role playing. Pitch pipe may be used to demonstrate sound. Teacher should stand behind the child so she cannot be seen and sound can be heard. Of course, older children do not require lengthy preparation.

IV. Description and use of audiometer

    A. Audiometer: Electronic instrument that measures hearing acuity suitable as screening device and accurate enough to establish necessity for referrals.

    B. Frequency control or pitch control: Obtained by frequency selector or oscillator, which creates tone.

    C. Cycles per second (CPS) = frequency: Lowest frequency audible is 125 CPS; middle C = 256 CPS; O = symbol for right ear; X = symbol for left ear.

    D. Screening technique: Quiet room—sound-treated acoustic tiled ceiling and plastic walls (when possible, this is ideal), drapes, carpeting, and shelves of books.

    E. Types of tests

        1. Individual pure tone "sweepcheck" screening test (Figs. 5-14 and 5-15) requires 30 to 45 seconds per child. Test 500, 1000, 2000, and 4000. Frequency level of intensity is decibels. Results vary. ASA—screen at 15 db; ISO—screen at 20 to 25 db.

        2. Decibel is slightest amount of intensity (sound pressure) change between frequencies audible to the human ear.

        3. 0db is slightest amount of intensity (sound pressure) required by the human ear to barely perceive a specific frequency.

        4. Conversation speech range 300 to 3000 CPS clarity.

    F. Criteria for referral

        1. Loss of 20 db in two frequencies in one ear

        2. Loss of 30 db in any frequency

        3. Slight or mild loss with evidence of pathology leading to hearing loss—for example, draining ear

V. Correlation

The area of hearing can be correlated in the following various subjects:

Arithmetic: Squares—solids.

Science and social studies: Units of study on care of ears.

Health: How well do we hear and the importance of a doctor's visit when the need arises.

Art: Tracing the ear diagram.

Music: The children like to play on toy musical instruments. Making musical instruments; experimenting on the tuning fork; and a xylophone.

Language arts: Having children write good health rules on the care of ears—vocabulary. Let children tell why they have ears. Talk about animal ears.

Show pictures of dog, cat, cow, and rabbit. Discuss how they use their ears for protection.

Safety: Discuss how to protect ears from loud noises; the danger of yelling in others' ears; of television or radio turned on loud; or of hitting others on ears. Discuss danger of pulling ears. Ask how a cat or dog reacts when we pull their ears. Have children write a class story about ears. Then have each one draw a picture to illustrate it.

VI. Hearing screening in public schools

Develop a good public relation with school personnel, superintendent, school board, teachers, and custodians.

A. Find a way to do follow-up.

B. Have the medical society endorse your program.

C. Get permission from school superintendent and go over your plans with him. Have answers to his questions.

    1. Why to test?

    2. Who to test?

    3. How long will it take?

    4. Where will the test be done, etc.?

D. After receiving permission, the nurse should give news release to the newspaper, radio, television, and Parent-Teacher Association. Nurse should also stress the importance of this test. Send letters to the medical staff and dental staff. Give them the plans in detail and see if they will accept referrals.

E. Planning stage will take approximately three weeks.

    1. Set dates with school, principal, and teachers.

    2. Survey building for the best place for screening and rooms for rechecks.

F. If money is involved, put a request for it in planning.

G. If permission slips are used, explain the program well but in short, easy, and understandable terms. Send slips home two weeks in advance, but never send consent slips home on Fridays.

H. Make a room list and check off as they return.

PROCEDURE SUMMARY

I. Who to test

A. Kindergarten, first, second, and fourth grades or first, third, and fourth grades.

B. Kindergarten, first, fourth, seventh, and eighth grades plus those with previously known hearing problems.

C. Teacher referrals—the following problems would help her decide which students to refer:

    1. Reading difficulties

    2. Speech problems

    3. Ear problems

    4. Those who do not understand assignments

    5. Those for whom the teacher must keep repeating the questions

    6. Those with a history of hearing problems

II. When to test

A. Do early in the day.

B. Do not test on holidays.

C. If the testing lasts all day, start with the younger children first.

D. Arrange testing with school schedule so that it is not at recess or noon.

III. Help needed

A. Have teachers list students and make out individual slips.

B. Parent-Teacher Association should be available to help. Use one person for each setup, to do rechecks, and to control traffic to and from room and to help to keep the noise down.

IV. Testing day

A. Give instructions to students in rooms as to the procedure.

B. Check name slips all made out in advance.

C. The tester will keep slips and mark as to the findings.

D. Give slips back to teacher on rechecks; keep others.

E. Pick a sharp student first if possible.

V. Rechecks

A. To be done in as quiet a room as possible.

B. Helper will bring child from room with slip and guide student to recheck room.

C. Test good ear first.

D. Keep the tester busy; do not waste time. Rechecks take more time than screening.

VI. Follow-up

A. An average of 5 percent need follow-up.

B. Send I.S.U. for pure tone testing if possible.

C. Refer to doctor.

D. Confer with parents, teachers, and principal to make them aware of those who did not pass the test and that they need further testing.

E. Money for follow-up when parent cannot pay

1. Department of public assistance

2. Health department

3. Civic organizations

PROCEDURES FOR PREVENTING DISEASE AND DEALING WITH EXISTING HEALTH PROBLEMS

Each child has the right to safe, effective care if sick or injured, and the same right to be protected from communicable disease by educational and preventive programs. Every child is distinct and separate in his abilities, interests, and potential and has a place in society where he can contribute to mankind. The school nurse's role in the special education of the handicapped child is related to her role in dealing with existing health problems and offers the greatest area of potential growth in expanding the nurse's responsibilities and contributions to the community.

By far the most common health problems of childhood are due to communicable diseases, which account for almost half of the absences from school. Therefore it is necessary to recognize signs and symptoms of illness that may be contagious and to isolate the child; in order to do this, nurses conduct clinics to prevent the outbreak of specific anticipated diseases. Based on statistical surveys, the needs and priorities of immunization clinics must be continually evaluated for all age groups.

Procedures for communicable disease control and policies for immunizations should be recommended by the local health department. Communicable disease control is constantly changing, and it is imperative that school nurses keep abreast of these changes and distribute this information to all those who come in contact with the schoolchild—other schoolchildren, counselors, teachers, office personnel, cooks, parents, custodians, and school bus drivers.

The procedures to be discussed in this section are as follows: communicable disease prevention immunization; communicable disease control; administration of prescription drugs; school nurses' role in special education of the handicapped; responsibilities of the school nurse in the program for educationally handicapped pupils; special services for partially sighted or blind; and students wearing glasses during physical education participation.

Communicable disease prevention immunization procedure

The prevention of communicable disease through provision of scientific up-to-date information regarding immunization to pupils, parents, and school personnel and the assurance of adequate immunization of all schoolchildren are important components of school health services.

I. Purpose

- A. To educate pupils, parents, and school personnel regarding the importance of adequate protection against disease by immunization
- B. To ensure adequate immunization of all schoolchildren
- C. To serve as a guide and reminder to parents for recommended boosters and revaccination

II. Procedure

- A. Plan with teachers and school administrators in each school for instruction in disease protection based on current community health projects, legal regulations, and specific school needs derived from records and reports.
- B. Assist in implementing the program by providing accurate information and resource materials in each school.
- C. Develop procedures with the administrators and teachers for keeping parents informed of current recommendations for disease protection and available sources for obtaining this protection.

D. Maintain up-to-date information on immunization status of all students in kindergarten or first grade and all pupils new to the district.

E. Send Disease Protection Reminder form any time the nurse is reviewing record and the need is indicated (Fig. 5-9).

III. Recording

A. Record available immunization information in the specified spaces on the existing Cumulative Record from such sources as the medical report, health inventory, health department certificates, and parent conferences or if information is available, place in Cumulative Record. EXCEPTION: See "C."

B. For senior high schools, information may be placed in the Cumulative Folder rather than be transcribed.

C. Record polio and measles immunizations in the most appropriate space of the existing health record.

Communicable disease control

Communicable disease control is an integral part of school health services. The school district follows current public health practices and rules and regulations governing the control and prevention of communicable diseases that are set up by the state department of public health and the health department.

I. Procedure

A. Communicable diseases

1. Interprets rules and regulations governing control and prevention of communicable disease to parents and school personnel.

2. Inspects pupils and school personnel with suspected communicable diseases and arranges for their exclusion.

3. Keeps school personnel informed regarding prevalent diseases and necessary control measures.

4. Provides administrators and elementary classroom teachers with a copy of rules and regulations governing communicable diseases.

5. Reports all *major* communicable diseases such as polio, meningitis, and active tuberculosis to the health department. This is done immediately for suspected or confirmed cases.

6. Works with school personnel in providing current scientific information for health instruction in control and prevention of communicable disease.

B. Nuisance diseases

Excludes all pupils suspected of the following diseases until condition is cleared or note is received from the family health adviser or clinic stating that the condition is under treatment and is controlled to the extent that pupil is not communicable to others:

1. Impetigo and ringworm of the skin

Pupils with inflamed lesions from impetigo and ringworm of the skin small enough to be covered may be kept in school if treatment is in progress and pupils are kept under observation. With oral medication, the lesions can often be uncovered in two to three days.

2. Ringworm of the scalp

    a. Inform parent of condition by telephone and note (Fig. 5-17).

    b. If three or more cases of ringworm of the scalp exist in a classroom, all pupils in the class should be inspected with the Woods lamp. These

---

SCALP CONDITION LETTER

Date_____

Dear Parent or Guardian:

Your child has been excluded from school because of a scalp condition which may be contagious.

In order that your child may return to school with as little loss of time as possible, will you please take him/her, at your earliest convenience, to your family health advisor for diagnosis.

Please have the family health advisor sign the lower portion of this blank and have the child bring it to the school upon his/her return.

DIRECTOR
Department of Health Services

_____
(Signature of Principal)

Date_____

To the Principal:

_____ was examined today and the scalp condition was
(Student's Name)
found to be:

☐   Non-contagious — may attend school.

☐   Contagious — this condition is under treatment and the child may attend school if the lesions are covered.

_____
(Signature of Family Health Advisor)

13-0161-01 11M155-1

Fig. 5-17. Scalp Condition Letter.

Pediculosis (lousiness)

I. Control measures

A. Control of infested person, contacts, and the immediate environment:
1. Report to local health authority: Official report not ordinarily justifiable.
2. Isolation: Not necessary after application of effective insecticide.
3. Concurrent disinfestation: Of other members of family or associated group.
4. Terminal disinfection: None.
5. Quarantine: None.
6. Immunization of contacts: Does not apply.
7. Investigation of contacts and source of infestation: Examination of household and other close personal contacts, with concurrent treatment as indicated.

B. Specific treatment: 10% DDT dusting powder for body and head lice; dust clothing, particularly along seams, and the hair; cover head with towel or cap for several hours; comb hair with fine-tooth comb, repeat dusting in one week without washing hair or clothing in the interim. For crab lice, dust hairy parts of body and bathe after twelve to twenty-four hours; repeat treatment in one week; continue treatment at weekly intervals until lice or nits are no longer present. Gamma isomer or benzene hexachloride (Lindane) as a 1% dusting powder or a 1% ointment, Kwell, may be substituted; is lethal to both lice and their eggs. Shampoo followed by application of 1% gamma benzene hexachloride in cream or lotion is effective and acceptable for head lice.

II. Description of disease

A. Identification: Infestation of the scalp, of the hairy parts of the body, or of clothing, especially along the seams of inner surfaces, with adult lice, larvae, or nits. Synonym: Lousiness.
B. Infesting agents: *Pediculus humanus,* head louse or body louse, and *Phthirus pubis,* crab louse. Animal lice do not infest man.
C. Reservoir and source of infestation: Reservoir is infested persons. Sources of infestation are such persons themselves and their personal belongings, particularly body clothing or infested bedding.
D. Mode of transmission: Direct contact with an infested person and indirectly by contact with clothing and headgear of such persons.
E. Incubation period: Under optimum conditions the eggs of lice hatch in a week, and sexual maturity is reached in approximately two weeks.
F. Period of communicability: While lice remain alive on the infested person or in his clothing, and until eggs (nits) in hair and clothing have been destroyed.
G. Susceptibility and resistance: Any person may become lousy under suitable conditions of exposure. Repeated infestations often result in dermal hypersensitivity.
H. Occurrence: Worldwide. The head louse is common in outbreaks among schoolchildren.

III. Nursing responsibilities

A. Urge medical examinations for suspects who present conditions described under Description of Disease and report school and institutional outbreaks to the respective authorities.

Pediculosis (lousiness)

III. Nursing responsibilities—cont'd

    B. Provide teachers and parents with information that will help them to recognize infestation. Instruct teachers and parents how to inspect heads with tongue blades, using separate sets for each person, and to dispose of used tongue blades in paper for burning.

    C. Collect specimens of infested hair for identification by Bureau of Vector Control when requested.

    D. Follow health department policy on excluding children from school. Teach infested individual and family to:

        1. Delouse head and body according to medical instructions.

        2. Wash infested person's clothing and bed linen with soap and hot water after treatment has been completed.

        3. Understand value of home and personal cleanliness.

        4. Use residual insecticide according to directions, but store insecticides out of reach of young children.

        5. Disinfest family or associated group concurrently to prevent reinfestation.

        6. Look for possible skin irritations from topical treatment and report them to the attending physician.

        7. Assist in finding additional infested persons among contacts.

    E. Participate in the education of individuals, and the general public when indicated, on modes of transmission and measures for preventing infestation as outlined under Control Measures above.

---

        lamps and instructions in their use are secured by the nurse through the central office.

    c. When possible, a note from the private physician or clinic permitting attendance should be secured.

    d. Pupils under treatment must wear suitable head covering when in school. In elementary schools this means a stocking cap.

  3. Pediculosis

    Pupils must be excluded until free of live nits. This problem is particularly difficult, since other members of the family are frequently infested and the pupil may become reinfested. The procedure concerning pediculosis (lousiness) (see material in box) is often helpful in informing parents of care and treatment.

  4. Scabies

    Pupils must be excluded until skin is clear or note from family health adviser indicates that treatment has controlled the infection.

II. Recording incidence of communicable disease

    A. The classroom teachers will record incidence of disease on the Cumulative Health Record as they occur in the classroom.

    B. The pupil's history of communicable disease is recorded on the Cumulative Health Record from medical or health inventory reports.

Administration of prescription drugs by school personnel

The Assembly Bill no. 1066, Chapter 681, State of California Education Code, includes the following provision:

> 11753.1 Notwithstanding the provisions of Section 11753, any pupil who is required to take, during the regular school day, medication prescribed for him by a physician, may be assisted by the school nurse or other designated school personnel if the school district received (1) a written statement from such physician detailing the method, amount and time schedules by which such medication is to be taken and (2) a written statement from the parent or guardian of the pupil indicating the desire that the school district assist the pupil in the matters set forth in the physician's statement.

This bill apparently permits rather than mandates the assistance of school personnel in administering drugs prescribed by a physician to pupils. This procedure should not be routine and should be implemented only when there is no other possible means of treatment.

I. Preliminary procedure

    A. The school nurse is responsible for the following steps:
        1. Ascertain directly from the physician treating the pupil that administering the medication at school is necessary for the health and well-being of the child and that no other time schedule for taking the drug is possible.
        2. Obtain a written statement from the doctor stating diagnosis, method and amount, and the time medication must be given.
        3. Obtain a written statement from the parent or guardian requesting that the school personnel assist the pupil as recommended by the doctor.
        4. Orders regarding changes in medication can be accepted by the school nurse via the telephone.

II. On-site school procedure

    A. The school nurse should develop an appropriate procedure with the principal at each school.
    B. Insofar as possible, plan with the parent and child so that pupil can administer his own drug if needed at school.
    C. Limit the amount of drugs kept at school.
    D. Keep medication in a safe place—away from other students in a locked cupboard.
    E. If medication is kept at school, use usual method of checking drug dosage at each administration at school.
    F. Keep an accurate record of each dose administered at school including date, time, and person giving medication (Fig. 5-18).

III. Follow-up procedure

If there is a daily dosage the school nurse should check with the attending physician at intervals no greater than every three months to determine the efficacy of the medication and if the drug needs to be continued at school.

RECORD OF THE ADMINISTRATION OF A PRESCRIPTION DRUG

_____

SCHOOL

CHILD'S NAME_____

Drug Order_____

Doctor_____

Date of Initial Order_____

Renewal Dates _____

DATE	TIME	AMOUNT	BY WHOM	COMMENTS

Fig. 5-18. Record of the Administration of a Prescription Drug.

School nurses' role in special education of the handicapped

School nurses are a part of professional teams employed to aid children and youth in developing their full potential in health and education. From their basic profession, nurses bring to their teams special knowledge and skills. Their unique contribution lies in their leadership ability to relate their particular understandings of nursing and health to the educational process and conditions that affect learning.

I. **Role and responsibility**

A. Some children need special understanding; some need special help from their parents or teacher; some need special classes.

B. These exceptional children are identified as follows:
1. Pupils with intellectual limitations
2. Pupils with superior intellect
3. Pupils with behavior problems
4. Pupils with speech problems
5. Pupils with impaired hearing
6. Pupils with impaired vision
7. Pupils with neurological and nonsensory physical impairments

C. Role of the school nurse in early identification of health problems
1. Health appraisal procedures
   a. Encourage families to provide for health examinations of their children by utilizing services of private physicians, dentists, and clinics.
   b. Develop procedures by which the findings and recommendations are reported to the school.
   c. Plan schedule for school health appraisal procedures with administrators, teachers, and other pupil personnel staff.
   d. Administer or arrange for screening procedures for all pupils:
      (1) Vision and hearing screening
      (2) Arrange for speech and language assessments
   e. Utilize health appraisal activities as educational experiences by:
      (1) Pupil preparation prior to all health appraisal procedures
      (2) Individual counseling during and following health appraisal activities
2. Follow-through procedures
   a. Interpret possible need of appraisal to parents.
   b. Encourage parents to initiate health conferences.
   c. Help parent obtain care through public and private community facilities and obtain financial aid when necessary.
   d. Obtain health history—obtain pertinent health information from private doctors, clinics, etc.; develop permission forms for the exchange of information.
   e. Interpret findings to administrative personnel, teachers, and parents:
      (1) Seek to have each child treated as nearly normal as possible.
      (2) Assist in developing plans for modification of educational programs where necessary:
         (a) Preferential seating for hearing or vision loss
         (b) Developing healthful school environment for the handicapped —appropriate desks, chairs, and other equipment, ramps, acoustics, etc.
         (c) Physical education modifications, rest periods when indicated
         (d) Part-time school
         (e) Transportation
         (f) Home and hospital instruction

(g) Arrange for medication when prescribed

(h) Plans for periodic review of such modifications

 f. Counsel with pupils to:

  (1) Interpret appraisal findings

  (2) Help pupil to accept personal responsibility for treatment

  (3) Understand modification of health practices

  (4) Impart basic health knowledge related to their problems

II. Evaluation

 A. Effect

  1. Did we see children become functional that had been lost?

  2. Note social adjustment and peer relationships.

  3. Did attendance improve?

  4. Did we meet parents' needs regarding health matters? How?

  5. Were we effective in presenting the health problem of each special child to the staff?

  6. Did we see evidence that parents gained interest in this child as a result of our counseling? Did the child gain interest in solving his problem?

 B. Effort

  1. What screening programs were carried out?

   a. Hearing

   b. Vision

   c. Immunization status

   d. Dental inspection

  2. Follow-up procedures

   a. Parent contacts

   b. Medical and clinic contacts

   c. Community resource contacts

  3. Record keeping

   a. Files on these special youngsters

   b. Do we have exchange of information with other special services personnel?

Responsibilities of the school nurse in the program for educationally handicapped pupils

The school nurse plays an important auxiliary role in the program for educationally hadicapped by working cooperatively with the principal, special teachers for educationally handicapped, and other auxiliary workers in the school. The nurse should assist in appraising the health status of pupils considered for admission in these classes and interpret finding and any other pertinent data regarding the child or his family to school and community personnel. As the program progresses, the nurse should continually contribute information regarding these pupils.

I. Developmental history

A. The nurse, nurse assistant, or guidance consultant may be responsible for obtaining developmental or medical summary when pupil is being considered for the program.

B. Since nurse's time for this program is limited, be sure there is a clear understanding that a reasonable amount of time be allowed for obtaining this information. Priorities should be set. Nurses should not accept new referrals in the last two weeks of school.

C. Nurses will proceed in contacting parents, initiating developmental history, or requesting medical summaries *only* after individual test reports are available and a conference with the guidance consultant indicates the parent understands the child is being considered for special education. Nurses or nurse assistants should not make the initial contact with the family but should assist in obtaining the summary of neurological or psychiatric reports.

D. Complete developmental history and medical summary on all candidates.

E. Submit developmental summary and current physical evaluation, if no more than a year old, to school physician for review and further work-up.

F. All applications are evaluated by an interdisciplinary admissions committee and recommendations for disposition are made by this group.

II. Medical reports

A. Obtain signed Authorization for Information Medical form (Fig. 5-11) from parent or guardian and authorization for school information to be sent to physician or clinic.

B. Include vision and hearing test reports and any follow-up on all students. Retest vision if last test is over one year old.

III. Data for/from source of medical care

A. The following information, if pertinent, should be included when medical reports are requested from physician or clinic (this may be sent in a separate letter):

1. Name and phone number of school nurse and/or guidance worker.
2. Brief statement that child is being considered for special education.
3. Behavior in classroom.
4. Achievement in relation to performance, for example, "average ability, working below grade level."
5. Attention span.
6. Noted reactions to medication, if prescribed.
7. Any additional information regarding the child or his family that might assist the physician in making an accurate appraisal.

B. Request decision regarding medical evaluation and future medical plans for child.

C. Refer to school physician if available any problems or difficulties in obtaining medical reports from physicians or clinics.

IV. Re-evaluation of pupils

A. Keep up-to-date health and family information on all pupils on Nurses' Follow-Up Record cards (Fig. 5-2, *C* and *D*).

B. Keep principal, teachers, and others informed of any changes in health or family status.

C. Prepare reports for yearly evaluations, as requested by the department of special education.

Special services for partially sighted or blind

A program of special instruction for the partially sighted is provided by most schools. Specially trained teachers offer selected instructional materials and techniques for pupils with severe visual handicaps that interfere with the pupil's education. Selected totally blind students may have services available to them through interdepartmental agreement or interschool district agreement.

I. Referral of students

A. Criteria for referral—all students with visual acuity of 20/70 or less after correction or students with better vision who have complicated problems. Pupils with progressive myopia, nystagmus, congenital glaucoma, or cataracts are possible candidates.

B. Financial assistance may be needed for a limited number of selected pupils.

C. Application is made on the basis of a report of an eye specialist.

D. Medical eligibility may be reviewed and approved by the school physician, if indicated, in selected cases.

E. Medical information concerning the applicant should be submitted on form for Reporting Visually Handicapped Children and Youth. Forms are available upon request. Copies of original forms are returned to the school nurse.

F. Assignment to the program for the partially sighted is made by the director of special education.

G. A central file record is set up in the administration building on each case. Identification cards are kept on all students in the health services office at individual school sites.

II. Nursing follow-up

A. Record information concerning application and medical report on Cumulative Health Record and Nurses' Follow-Up Record card.

B. Send original eye examination report and Request for Special Service form to the department of health services for review and referral to the department of special education.

C. Obtain recheck report each calendar year from eye examiner.

D. Nurses will be notified if reports are *not* needed. Exceptions are cases on which a longer interval before recheck seems indicated.

E. Copies of reports are returned to the school nurse.

F. All reports not previously submitted are due in December.

G. Exchange pertinent information with teacher of partially sighted.

H. Keep Cumulative Health Record and Nurses' Follow-Up Report up to date.

I. Interpret to parents and pupils the program for the partially sighted and required annual reporting for financial information for the program.

J. Discuss the need for maintaining the best possible general health to enable the student to achieve to capacity.

III. Requests for release

Requests for release from the program for the partially sighted are recommended by the student's eye physician. Assignment is changed by the director of special education.

Students wearing glasses during physical education participation

I. All students wearing breakable-type glasses participating in the normal physical education program are required to wear eyeglass protectors. They shall not be permitted to participate unless they have such protection.

II. All students wearing either shatterproof plastic lenses or contact lenses may participate in the normal physical education program without eyeglass protection, provided the school has on file a statement from the students' parents or guardians giving permission to play without eyeglass protection.

III. Students who normally wear glasses but whose vision loss is not great enough to constitute a hazard in physical education activities when glasses are not worn may play without glasses.

IV. Physical education teachers should refer to the nurse the few students about whom there is some question as to the need for wearing glasses during physical education participation.

V. There may be cases where needy students may not be able to purchase protectors. In this instance, if the school wishes, it may purchase them out of funds now set aside for needy students.

CARE OF EMERGENCIES IN SCHOOLS

First aid care has changed and will continue to change over the years. All school personnel should have an up-to-date basic course in first aid for emergencies and be able to recognize signs or symptoms that might be indicative of a beginning communicable disease. Any individual of the school staff should be able to assess the situation and then:

1. Administer emergency care as needed.

2. Inform responsible people (principal, family member, or the person designated by the parent).

3. Refer to appropriate medical authority (family doctor, hospital, or police emergency squad).
4. As a matter of good public relations, the nurse or principal should make a follow-up contact with a family member within twenty-four hours with reference to final disposition of an accident or illness.
5. Record as needed on the health record. (The adoption of the accident form and accident-summary form as recommended by the National Safety Council is urged.)
6. Evaluate
   a. Could this accident have been prevented? How?
   b. Suggested ways of prevention sent to proper health authority if indicated to implement change as needed.
7. Specific guidelines for emergency care
   a. All school personnel should know basic first-aid procedures.
   b. A minimum of three people, skilled in the administration of first aid, should be available in *all* school buildings or areas of activities at all times.
   c. Emergency first-aid supplies should be kept in an easily accessible location that is known to all. Soap and water and dry sterile dressings may be kept in individual classrooms in the elementary and junior high schools.
   d. Emergency information card
   Appropriate current emergency data for all pupils and school personnel as provided by parent or individual shall be kept in a special, easily accessible file in each school.
   In the event the pupil does not know his telephone number and the number is not on record and is also unlisted, ask the operator to contact the family.

The first aid and emergencies procedure has been reviewed by the Child Welfare Committee of the Medical Association, and their suggestions have been included in this material. The procedure is set up in the following fashion for easy reference and use by all school personnel.

FIRST AID AND EMERGENCIES—GENERAL INFORMATION

RESPONSIBILITY OF THE SCHOOL	The responsibility of the schools for the health and physical well-being of pupils includes not only the time pupils are in attendance at school but also one hour before the opening of school and one hour after the closing of school.
EMERGENCY CARD	Appropriate, current emergency data for all pupils, provided by the parents, shall be kept in a special, easily accessible file at each school site.
RESPONSIBILITY FOR NOTIFYING PARENTS IN EMERGENCIES	The principal, his representative, or the nurse shall contact the parents or person designated to act in an emergency to arrange for removal of an ill or injured student from the school. The student is not permitted to leave school alone unless specifically authorized by the parent or person designated by parent. If necessary, a member of the school may take the pupil home or to a hospital when the condition does not require an ambulance.

In an accident the form Report of Accident to Pupil or Employee is completed according to instructions on the blank. In case of suspected drug abuse or other serious conditions, the school principal should be informed, followed by a memo giving the nurse's assessment and subsequent follow-up. Nurse should retain duplicate copy.

EMERGENCY
TREATMENT
FACILITIES

Emergency service at a specified hospital is provided for persons seriously ill or severely injured at school. Medical care at the emergency center is limited to control of hemorrhage, alleviation of pain, treatment for shock and respiratory distress, treatment for poisoning, drug abuse, and splinting of fractured bones. Patients are then referred to their own doctor or clinic for further care. Patients who qualify or whose condition makes it necessary may remain in the hospital. The superintendent of the hospital has authority to sign permission for lifesaving measures when parent or guardian cannot be reached. Patients with other conditions are not treated at the emergency center but are interviewed and referred to their own doctor or clinic.

AMBULANCE

1. In cases requiring an ambulance, the police department should be contacted by the school principal through his secretary. The patient will be taken to the city hospital unless directed otherwise. There is a charge to the family. Welfare families can be reimbursed for this charge.

   If the family wishes to use a hospital other than one specified, they should first contact their doctor. The parent, or responsible adult, should accompany the child in the ambulance or meet him at the emergency center. In some instances it may be advisable for school personnel to accompany the child to the source of care until parent contact is made. The ambulance driver's report form should be signed by the parent, responsible adult, or the police—*not by the school personnel.*

2. In exceptional cases, such as diabetes, written directions filed at the school by the parent designating the specific hospital and naming the physician in charge of the case may be honored. Notify the doctor and hospital.

3. For injuries incurred during practice or games in interscholastic sports, request the ambulance driver to go to the emergency clinic at the hospital that is designated by the team member's athletic insurance policy.

NOTIFICATION TO
SUPERINTEN-
DENT'S OFFICE

The superintendent's office and health services office are to be notified by telephone whenever an ambulance is summoned:

EMERGENCY CARE FOR STUDENTS FILING MEDICAL EXEMPTION CARDS

If the parents of the pupil have filed a Christian Science exemption card with the school, the following procedure should be followed:

1. Minor injuries, such as small cuts and abrasions, should be washed with plain soap and water only.
2. If the injury requires more than the above, the parent should be contacted. No additional first aid should be given.
3. If lifesaving measures are indicated and the parents cannot be reached, the student should be taken to the emergency hospital.

SEVERE INJURIES (GUNSHOT WOUNDS, STAB WOUNDS, ETC.)

1. Do not attempt to move patient.
2. Secure open airway.
3. If patient is not breathing spontaneously, give mouth-to-mouth resuscitation or insert airway and begin mouth-to-mouth resuscitation until the ambulance arrives.
4. Check for bleeding. Use sterile gauze pressure dressings to control bleeding. Use tourniquets to help control bleeding only if appropriate and as a last resort.
5. Treat for shock. Keep patient warm with blankets and keep constant check on pulse and respiration.
6. Remain with patient until ambulance arrives. Delegate others to call ambulance, notify principal of school, notify parents, bring blankets and first-aid supplies.

PROCEDURE FOR HUDSON AIRWAYS

1. Place victim on his back.
2. From behind the patient, lift the chin and tilt the head backward as far as possible.
3. Force mouth open slightly so the tube can be inserted. Use large end for adults, small end for children over 3 or 4 years old. If foreign matter is visible, clear the mouth and throat by rolling head to one side and sweeping fingers through the throat.
4. Slide tube through teeth and over the tongue until flange touches and seals lips.
5. Pinch nose closed with thumbs using other fingers to *keep chin up, head back,* and *lips closed.*
6. Blow air into tube until chest rises. Remove your mouth, allow patient to breathe out. Repeat every four to five seconds until revival. If chest movement is not noticed, readjust tube and try again.

MEDICATIONS

Any form of medication, including aspirin, should not be administered by school personnel to pupils. EXCEPTION: Prescription drugs, see special procedure implementing this in Section 11753.1 of the California Education Code for administering prescription drugs. (See p. 84.)

ABDOMINAL PAIN

Severe pain with or without nausea or fever
1. Notify parent or guardian and refer to family's usual source of medical care.
2. Keep child quiet in bed.
3. Do not give food or liquid.
4. Advise parents not to give laxative, enema, or suppository.

ABRASIONS AND CUTS

Superficial skin injuries (abrasions, cuts, and scratches)
1. Clean with liquid or bar soap and water.
2. Apply adhesive bandage or dry gauze dressing when needed.
Deep or extensive wounds
1. Control bleeding with sterile gauze dressing applied firmly to site.
2. Refer child to parents or responsible adult and family's usual source of medical care.
3. Do not move unnecessarily.
Puncture wounds
1. Allow to bleed freely.
2. Wash with liquid soap.
3. Apply sterile gauze dressing.
4. Advise parent to consult their usual source of medical care if there is contamination which might cause lockjaw (tetanus).

BITES

Dog bites
1. Notify parent and the police department. Give all possible identifying information about dog. Retain animal if possible.
2. Flush wound with large amounts of water. Cleanse with liquid or bar soap and water.
3. Apply sterile gauze dressing.
4. Urge parent to notify and consult the family's source of medical care.
Human bites
1. Cleanse wound with liquid or bar soap and water.
2. Apply sterile gauze dressing.
3. Urge parent to seek medical attention in all cases.
Insect bites such as bee stings, wasp bites, and spider bites
1. Remove stinger if possible.
2. Apply cold compresses.
3. Depending on type of bite and reaction, notify parent and/or refer to family medical adviser.
Other warm-blooded animal bites
1. Follow same procedure as for dog bites.
Snake bites
1. Nonpoisonous
   a. Treat as for puncture wound.
   b. Notify parent and refer to medical care as indicated.

2. Poisonous
   a. Keep patient as quiet as possible.
   b. Apply cold (preferably ice packs) to area to reduce blood circulation in the area. Mild restriction of return flow of blood from area by pressure may also be used. Application of ice pack must be alternated with period of natural warming of area.
   c. Notify parent.
   d. Take child to hospital.

BURNS
1. Immerse in cold water.
2. If skin is only reddened or has small blisters, apply sterile gauze dressing. Do not open blisters.
3. For more severe burns, cover with nonadhesive sterile gauze dressing or plastic film (household plastic wrap) without ointment and refer to parent and family medical adviser.
4. Burns caused by chemicals should be washed immediately with large quantities of clean water and treated as in 2.

DIABETIC COMPLICATIONS (INSULIN REACTION)
1. Obtain individual orders on all diabetic children.
2. Signs of insulin reaction such as paleness, sweating and trembling or shakiness, headache, feeling of faintness, unusual hunger, nausea, blurring of vision, confusion, or peculiar behavior should be treated by giving fruit juice, sugar, or candy immediately.
3. Notify parents if symptoms persist, or student may be taken home.
4. If reaction is severe (unconsciousness or convulsions), obtain *immediate medical care.*

DRUG ABUSE
1. Students who are stuporous to unconscious and little or no response can be elicited:
   a. Do not take time to ascertain type of drug or amount taken.
   b. Notify the principal immediately and, if alone, request assistance of another adult.
   c. Call police ambulance following the established routine.
   d. Make every effort to reach the parent.
2. Students who demonstrate abnormal behavior and are unable to function normally in a classroom situation, but whose vital signs are not indicative of any immediate danger:
   a. Notify the principal and, if alone, request assistance of another adult.
   b. Make every effort to notify the parent and recommend appropriate medical care.
   c. If the parent cannot be reached, refer to the principal or a person designated by him for follow-up decisions.

3. Follow usual procedure for reporting serious accidents or sudden illness to the superintendent's office and health services.

4. Reporting to the police is solely the responsibility of the principal of the school.

DYSMENORRHEA (MENSTRUAL CRAMPS)

1. Patient may lie down.
2. Apply blanket if desired.
3. Refer to physician if there are frequent recurrences of severe degree.

EARS

Earache

1. Take temperature.
2. Exclude and refer to parent and family's usual source of medical care.
3. Do not put anything into the ear.

Discharging ears

1. Refer parent to family medical adviser.
2. Allow free drainage. Do not use cotton plugs in ears.

Foreign body in ear or nose

1. Do not try to remove foreign body unless this procedure is simple.
2. Refer to parent and family's usual source of medical care.

EYES

Foreign body in eye

1. Instruct child not to rub eye. Have him close it gently, in the hope that the tears may wash the speck out or into view. If feasible, wash eye with clear water.
2. If foreign body remains and can be seen on the white of the eye, it may be removed with the corner of a sterile gauze pad.
3. If not easily removed, cover eye with dry gauze dressing and refer immediately to parent and family medical adviser.

Chemical burn to eye

1. Wash immediately and thoroughly with large quantities of tap water. Patient may be instructed to hold face under faucet or drinking fountain with eye open.
2. After above, refer immediately to parent and family's usual source of medical care. This condition *must* be seen by a physician for further care.

Eye wounds

1. Apply sterile gauze dressing.
2. Notify parent and refer to family's usual source of medical care.

Inflamed or discharging eyes

1. Exclude. Notify parent and refer to family's usual source of medical care.

FAINTING OR FEELING FAINTNESS

1. Fainting can often be prevented by having patient lie down or sit down with knees spread apart and head between knees.
2. Fainting—lay flat, cover with blanket. Children recover from

fainting rather promptly but should rest for thirty minutes to one hour after recovery.

3. Inhalation of spirits of ammonia may be used for the child who faints or feels faint. Avoid holding ammonia too close to nose.
4. Notify parent that faintness or fainting has occurred.
5. If above measures are used and patient has not recovered, obtain medical care immediately.

FEVER
1. If temperature is 99.6° F. or over without symptoms, exclude and refer to family's usual source of medical care.

FRACTURES
1. Support injured parts as may be necessary to prevent further injuries.
2. Unless position is unsafe, do not move patient until advised by a medically trained authority.
3. Keep patient warm and quiet.
4. If skin is broken, apply sterile gauze dressing.
5. In case of dental injury urge parents to obtain immediate dental attention. Advise against sharp changes in temperature (ice cream, hot and cold drinks) until first-aid treatment has been instituted by dentist.
6. Notify parent and refer to family's usual source of medical or dental care.

HEADACHES
1. Take temperature. If elevated, exclude child from school.
2. Rest in quiet room with fresh air.
3. Cold compresses on head may be used for comfort.
4. If severe and persistent, notify parent and refer to usual source of medical care.

HEAD INJURIES
A blow to any part of the head may produce only a momentary period of unconsciousness or a dazed condition and, following quick recovery, a headache is the only complaint. It is a mistake to assume that a rather prompt recovery from a dazed state is an indication that there is no serious injury. After a varying period of time, hours or days, the injured person may become drowsy or confused as a result of a brain injury. The following precautions should be taken:

1. If unconsciousness, convulsions, bleeding, or fluid from ears occur, notify parent and advise immediate medical care by direct transportation of the child to the hospital—not home and then to the hospital. If parent cannot be reached, use "transportation to emergency hospital" procedure.
2. If severe headache, nausea, vomiting, incoherence, drowsiness, or dazed appearance occurs, keep child at rest until parent is contacted for arrangements for medical care. Do not permit child to go home alone that day even if symptoms have disappeared.

3. For blows to the head not accompanied by any of the symptoms listed above:

   a. Allow child to rest for at least thirty minutes.

   b. Observe for symptoms noted above.

   c. Caution against overactivity.

   d. Notify parents of the blow to the head by telephone or by note sent home with the child.

   e. Make arrangements so that child will not walk home alone that day.

HEART ATTACK OR STROKE

1. Call ambulance service.
2. Notify person designated by parent or staff personnel.
3. Remain or have designated person remain with patient until ambulance arrives.

NAUSEA AND/OR VOMITING

1. Exclude child from school. Advise parent that if symptoms persist, refer to family's usual source of medical care.

NOSEBLEEDS

1. Have the patient sit with head tilted slightly back and breathing through mouth.
2. Press nostrils together for at least five minutes.
3. Apply cold compresses to nose if desired.
4. Avoid blowing nose for at least an hour.
5. Refer to parent and family's usual source of medical care for persistent or heavy bleeding.

POISON OAK

1. For relief of itching, apply cold compress or calamine lotion.
2. If lesions are severe or weeping, exclude and refer to parent and family medical adviser for care.
3. For recent exposure, wash thoroughly with soap and water.

POISON TAKEN INTERNALLY

1. Administer universal antidote (Res-Q), following directions on label or have patient drink four to seven glasses of water of milk.
2. Notify parent.
3. Secure immediate medical attention.

SEIZURE DISORDERS

Grand mal or convulsive seizure

1. Ease pupil to the floor and loosen collar. Do not try to restrain the jerking.
2. Turn head to one side for easy release of saliva and place some padding under head for comfort.
3. Move away furniture and hard objects that he might strike while jerking.
4. It is not necessary to put something between teeth.
5. Assign someone to watch the patient until jerking stops. The other members of the class should continue with class instruction as in any other medical emergency.

6. Do not try to revive with fluids, stimulants, fresh air, or walking.
7. After jerking has ceased, a small child can be carried to a rest room until ready to resume activity, and a large one allowed to lie until able to walk.
8. Notify parent. When attack is over, child who is on medication for the disorder may continue with his school schedule unless parent requests otherwise. If it is a known epileptic case, it is not usually necessary to call a doctor immediately.
9. Judgment with regard to disposition must be individualized for each child.
10. No accident report is necessary for an uncomplicated seizure —but only when pupil may have received some physical injury as from a fall.
11. Allow patient to rest quietly thirty minutes or more after attack.

SKIN CONDITIONS

Scabies, impetigo, ringworm, pediculosis
1. Exclude and refer to parent and family medical adviser for diagnosis and treatment.

Secondary skin infection and boils
1. Do not treat.
2. May cover with dry sterile gauze dressing and refer to parent.

SORE THROATS
1. If temperature is elevated or child appears ill, isolate and refer to parent and family medical adviser.

SPLINTERS
1. Wash area with soap and water.
2. Remove splinters with sterile tweezers if not deeply embedded.
3. Apply sterile gauze dressing if needed.
4. If deeply embedded, refer to parent and family medical adviser.

SPRAINS AND BRUISES
1. Elevate and support sprained area.
2. Do not tape or splint.
3. Refer to parent and family medical adviser.

TOOTHACHES
1. Temporary relief: swab cavity with cotton applicator saturated with oil of cloves or eugenol.

First-aid supplies

First-aid supplies are required for all elementary classrooms, class excursions, and special areas in secondary schools in order to provide immediate care for all minor injuries. Students with serious injuries should remain at the site of the accident until professional assistance is available.

I. Teacher first-aid kits

> 25 adhesive bandages
> 1 package of applicators
> 1 bottle of liquid soap

II. Class excursion first-aid kits

> 25 adhesive bandages
> 1 package of applicators
> 1 bottle of liquid soap
> 1 pair of blunt scissors (from general school supplies)
> 6 sterile gauze pads, 3 × 3 inches
> 2 gauze roller bandages, 2 inch
> 4 triangular bandages
> 1 roll of adhesive tape, ½ inch wide (10 yards)
> 1 first-aid instruction for use of content of first-aid kit (either a copy of the "First Aid and Emergencies Administrative Bulletin 14," Revised November, 1965, or a *Red Cross First-Aid Book*)
> 3 ampuls aromatic spirits of ammonia

A snake bite kit should be requisitioned from the warehouse when the school feels the need for one.

III. Supplies for special areas within the school

> (School shops, laboratories, cafeterias, homemaking, arts and crafts, gymnasium, etc.)
> 1 bottle of liquid soap
> 1 box of applicators (box of 72)
> 1 box of adhesive bandages (box of 25)
> 1 roll of adhesive tape, ½ inch wide
> 1 box of sterile gauze squares, 3 × 3 inches (box of 25)
> 1 bandage, 2 inches wide
> 1 package of paper eyecups for eye irrigation
> 1 pair of blunt scissors

SUMMARY MODEL

GUIDE FOR THE SCHOOL HEALTH PROGRAM

Name of school_____ Name of principal_____

Number of teachers_____ Number of pupils_____ Grades_____

Date this form completed_____ By_____

(Complete at principal-nurse conference or at faculty meeting. See that all school personnel and ancillary personnel receive final copies of this.)

1. School nursing time in the school
   Schedule

2. Facilities
   Where will the school nurse work?

   What telephone will be convenient to use?

   How are supplies requested?

3. Health information and examinations
   How is information on health, including health inventories, medical, and dental reports, obtained?

   For routine grades?

   For special health problems?

4. Accidents and emergency illness
   Is the school oriented to approved first-aid policies?

   Are these policies approved by the medical association and the health department and adopted by the board of education?

   When will the school nurse demonstrate and interpret these policies at a faculty meeting?

GUIDE FOR THE SCHOOL HEALTH PROGRAM—CONT'D

How will the first-aid cupboard be maintained and supplies ordered during the year?

Who will give first aid and care for emergency illnesses—school secretary, nurse assistant, individual teachers, principal—when the nurse is at another school? How does the school contact a nurse in case of severe accident or illness?

What records are kept?

Is there a plan for analyzing the causes of accidents in line with accident prevention?

5. Conferences
Principal-nurse conference
How can the school nurse best keep the principal informed?

When would it be possible to schedule planned conferences?

How will schedule be set up?

How should informal conferences be arranged?

Multiple disciplinary conferences
How should conferences be arranged with the school psychologist, speech therapist, and/or teacher and parent regarding a specific pupil?

Should the principal always be notified and included?

6. Plan for referral of students for follow-up
How are pupils whose health appears to deviate from normal referred to the nurse?

GUIDE FOR THE SCHOOL HEALTH PROGRAM—CONT'D

How should teacher request services of the school nurse?

How are medical referrals made? By the teacher, principal, nurse, or a combination of any of these?

How do referrals by others get back to the nurse?

Are there any medical referrals the principal wants to be informed of?

How should the school be informed of outcomes of referrals?

What procedure is followed for the school for referral for psychological testing or the services of the guidance consultant?

What procedure is followed for referral to special education?

7. Vision screening program
   What would be the best time to schedule vision screening?

   What arrangements are made to make this program on educational experience in the classroom?

   Who will record test results on school health records—nurses, teachers, and nurse assistants?

8. Hearing program
   Have dates been set for hearing testing?

   Date school is scheduled for testing _____.
   What arrangements are made to make this an educational experience in the classroom?

GUIDE FOR THE SCHOOL HEALTH PROGRAM—CONT'D

What provisions are available for special education recommendations—desk amplifiers, speech correction, etc.?

9. Communicable disease control
   Immunizations
   How is information to be obtained on new students?

   How is the immunization status of all students kept up to date?

   How are parents or students informed when immunizations are needed?

   Exclusions and admissions
   Is the guide regarding exclusions and admissions for communicable disease approved by the health department available at the school site?

10. Dental health
    Can the school nurse be of assistance in planning dental health education programs?

    Does the teacher make use of dental visual aids in teaching dental health education in the classroom?

    Are pupils encouraged to have regular dental checkups?

    Are pupils excused from school for dental appointments?

    Does the teacher refer pupils with obvious dental defects to the nurse for follow-up and encourage pupils to report to her conditions of the mouth that disturb them?

    Are school personnel aware of recommended first-aid procedures to follow in case of dental emergencies—fractured jaw, broken teeth, etc.?

GUIDE FOR THE SCHOOL HEALTH PROGRAM—CONT'D

Is the school aware of how to procure emergency funds, if available?

11. Nutrition
How should school personnel request nutrition information and consultation from the school nurse?

Do the majority of the pupils use the school breakfast and lunch program?

Are observations made of pupil's nutritional practices to stimulate improvement through instruction?

Are spot observations made on contents of home-packed lunches?

12. Health instruction
Can the school nurse be of help by providing up-to-date factual information to help in classroom health projects?

Will requests come through the principal or directly from the teachers?

How should the nurse bring to the attention of the school information regarding specific health problems of the community or among the pupils who may need educational emphasis?

Is there a school health council?

Who is the representative?

Is there a student health council?

Who plans the programs?

GUIDE FOR THE SCHOOL HEALTH PROGRAM—CONT'D

13. Faculty meetings
Which faculty meetings should the nurse plan to attend?

14. Parent-Teacher Association—parent groups
Is there a Parent-Teacher Association or parent group in the school?

Who is the president for this year? What is her address and telephone number?

Who is the health chairman for this year? What is her address and telephone number?

Is the nurse invited to attend meetings?

Is it a source for volunteer help for school or community health programs?

Who contacts these groups for assistance?

15. Records
Discuss procedure for routing health information, medical reports, etc.

Does the teacher or counselor know of the Cumulative Health Record maintained by the school on each pupil and what information is recorded on it?

Who are school personnel responsible for recording information on the school Cumulative Health Record?

EVALUATION
1. Objectives of the school health program this year:

2. What are suggestions for improvement?

6

SCHOOL NURSING PRACTICE

HEALTH EDUCATION

Health education means many things to many people, but in school nursing practice it encompasses all the health teaching performed by the nurse. This includes individual and group counseling on physical, social, and mental health and preparation with others of health curriculum, classroom instruction, and parent and teacher education.

Health counseling

Health counseling is undoubtedly the most important skill of the school nurse and must be based on the principle of democratic leadership. In counseling, nurses show respect for the individual personality and a feeling of understanding or empathy. Of course it is important that the nurse possesses the knowledge of health and the skill to perform this activity. The nurses who like their work usually have a positive attitude and demonstrate sincere, enthusiastic interest to inspire learning. Pupils, teachers, or parents respond best when one is interested in their problems and when the nurse will listen, discuss the problem, and consider suggestions for adjustment. People need a degree of love, warmth, praise, and consistency.

Health counseling may be done in various ways. The typical setting is arranged in the nurse's office to meet with the individual child, groups of children, parent, or groups of parents and/or teachers. Health counseling may require larger space than the nurse's office, such as a classroom or the multipurpose room, if a group wants counseling on a certain topic of interest to all members. A common setting for health counseling is in the homes of parents. Nurses must determine the best environment for what they need to accomplish.

One factor in health counseling is acceptance of one another. How is the nurse accepted by the individual or group? Then, too, how does the nurse accept this individual or group of individuals? We speak of this in the interview setting as a condition of harmony or rapport, which can be the crux of the whole health counseling setting.

Health problems are sometimes solved by careful scrutiny and using the scientific method of approach. This can be done by simply asking questions such as the following:

1. *What* is the problem? Can you state it as you find it to be?
2. *How* does this affect the individual? How does it affect the family, the classroom, the community?

3. *Why* do we discuss this problem?
   a. What do you think will solve the problem?
   b. Can you make a tentative plan to correct the problem?
4. *Results* can be interpreted in what manner?
   a. What are the results of the attempt for correction of the problem?
   b. What did you learn from the way you handled this problem?

Helping children, parents, and teachers explore their own areas of concern can be a satisfying experience for all people involved.

Health instruction

The National Education Association and the American Medical Association long ago defined health instruction as "the organization of learning experiences directed toward the development of favorable health knowledges, attitudes, and practices." The result of instruction is a change in behavior.

There is seldom a time when all children in the same class are at the same stage of growth. Each child is an individual with his own maturation rate. So the school nurse in preparing health instruction considers signs of growth and development in terms of physical, intellectual, social, and emotional behavior. The following points are considered:

1. Laws of learning apply to health.
2. Motivation to learn influences behavior.
3. Interests and needs influence learning.
4. Pupil readiness to learn.
5. Teaching positively what to do.
6. Repetition of concepts with different approaches.
7. Rewards are superior to punishment.
8. Socializing promotes retention and recall.

Interests vacillate according to the school and community happenings. How can teachers and nurses plan for pupil readiness or determine their interests? By observation and communication one can evaluate children's interests; the following list suggests areas the nurse can observe to determine interests:

1. Talking to children
2. Listening to children talk with others
3. Watching what children do
   a. Before school
   b. After school
   c. At play
   d. During unassigned periods
4. Evaluating children's expressions and activities
   a. Drawings
   b. Crafts
   c. Stories
   d. How they express themselves to peers
5. Noticing their choices they share from home
   a. Books
   b. Stories and magazines

   c. Hobbies
   d. Care of pets
6. Parent conference
   a. What interests does this child have at home?
   b. What interests are shared as a family?

Micro health units

Micro health units integrate health education into the general school curriculum. This method does not replace the ongoing health education, but it adds impact to the learning process and interrelates health to general living.

The most important ingredient in the presentation of a micro unit is its pertinence to other learnings in the classroom. It takes a certain amount of research whereby the nurse or teacher is able to bring to the classroom a special emphasis in health education that can influence the students' knowledge and attitudes toward health. The nurse or teacher must ascertain the following:

1. The scope and sequence of classroom program and decide the best time to implement health teaching
2. That materials are appropriate to the grade level
3. That the lesson can be built on existing knowledge and a health concept can be generated from the material

The micro health units available explore social studies at various grade levels and present a health focus:

GRADE	SOCIAL STUDIES	MICRO HEALTH UNIT
2	Community helpers	Health services
3	Indians	Native plants and drugs
4	Japan—Africa	Comparative nutrition
5	Civil War	War-time medical conditions (then and now)
6	South America	Sanitation and infection

A further reference for the micro health units was made through the Rosenberg Foundation Grant and implemented at the Novato, California, Unified School District by Margaret Feldstein and Linda Swaab. Their series was used in Mt. Diablo Unified School District, Concord, California, and includes the following topics*:

California: Indian Garden of Eden
The Search for the Chain of Gold
Health Conditions on the Mayflower
Africa Health and Disease—Man
The State of Medicine at Valley Forge
World Food Challenges—Man, His Environment and the Future
Sugar and Spice and the F.D.A.
Puritan Land of Plenty—Food and Medicine in Colonial America

The team approach

Problems in the school deserve a team approach to be effectively solved, and sometimes parents are a part of this team. It is the responsibility of the administrative

*From Feldstein, Margaret, and Swaab, Linda: Micro health units, Rosenberg Foundation Grant, Novato, Calif., 1971.

personnel to keep teachers up-to-date on new programs and materials available to teachers that can be used in solving school problems. An in-service program is a helpful plan in dispersing such information.

Attention to the physical and mental health status of a faculty and the school team can be an ongoing project to challenge the imagination of the school admin-

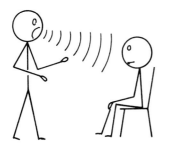

To discuss is not to lecture or to tell. Discussion is not a one-way process.

Discussion begins with a two-way exchange, e.g., the teacher questions; a student responds; the teacher comments.

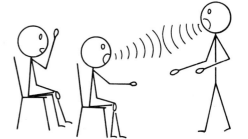

Discussion reaches its maximum effectiveness when there is interaction in many directions, e.g., the teacher questions; a student responds; a second student challenges the response; the first student defends his position; a third student asks a probing question; a fourth student suggests an alternative response; the teacher asks a fifth student if he agrees; and so on.

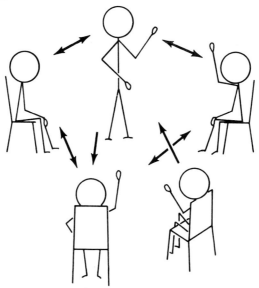

Fig. 6-1. Discussion and interactions.

istration. It is a well-known fact that we teach by example. A healthy teacher and healthy interrelationships displayed by the school team can be the most effective teaching method available to teach how to solve problems.

Parent education. More and more emphasis is placed on the education of parents in order to guide their children. Study groups and seminars are effective. Parents are usually questioned as to their needs. The most popular topics are discipline, drug abuse, promiscuity, and venereal disease, and often other specialists within the school or community are called upon to lead these groups. Fig. 6-1 is an interesting illustration of the discussion method and interactions.

Teacher participation. Teachers are in the key position to make a wholesome contribution to the health education of schoolchildren. Without their enthusiasm and understanding, a health program will not succeed, even though in many states health instruction is mandated by law. The physical health status of classroom teachers is related to their personal health practices. Teaching demands much vigor and enthusiasm of the individual; and teachers need diversion, play, and relaxation; hobbies can afford diversion. A healthy teacher is a good model for pupils.

Teachers should not overestimate pupils' knowledge of basic facts. It may be necessary to take a survey of the class to determine their basic knowledge and then to supplement the class curriculum with enrichment programs to inspire health in everyday living. Of course the environment is important for learning, and the teacher is responsible for the physical aspects as well as for the psychological climate of the classroom.

Conferences are held between the teacher and school nurse, and together referrals may be made for follow-up care as well as planning for health instruction. School health offices usually have health education media readily available to teachers. If not, nurses usually know sources of health materials that can be borrowed, made, or ordered.

Health can be taught by integrating its materials into other subjects as described in the micro health units where social studies was the core curriculum. The effectiveness of health education will be increased when it is so enriched. The curriculum has to be subject to change, yet the teacher needs guidelines, and the material taught should be scientifically sound.

Pupil participation. Physical fitness is a natural adjunct to health. So it is necessary for students to gain an understanding of how a proper balance of exercise, work, sleep, rest, and relaxation will provide physical and mental well-being. Implementing the health curriculum will afford an opportunity for pupils to experience meaningful, suitable activities to learn hygienic practices. Individual differences in a classroom must be considered, but the activities to promote better understanding of health depend on pupil participation, imagination, and creativity.

An example of a quick motivating device is the game of a sectioned wheel with a spinning indicator pointing to the section to be discussed. The sections of the wheel represent the personal needs and interests, which the class had previously decided upon, such as cleanliness, exercise, sleep and rest, dental health, food and eating, safety, clothing, emotional adjustments, and other areas, depending on the enthusiasm of classroom participation and on the grade level. This quick device may be used for inspections and to get responses from children because everyday they must be prepared for the area indicated for discussion. The game creates a habit for good daily healthful living, and the children have fun spinning the wheel. By using this habitual daily device a teacher is able to detect deficiencies in health care and can assist children in evaluating themselves.

The following list suggests ways that pupils may participate in a health curriculum:

1. Make displays
2. Prepare reports
3. Share on committee work
4. Make surveys
5. Show films and make their own films
6. Show film strip and discuss its contents
7. Prepare charts
8. Prepare posters
9. Share in an animal experiment (nutrition)
10. Provide pamphlets, books, newspaper articles on topics of interest
11. Dramatize topic
12. Role play
13. Debates
14. Plan local excursion to identify community or outdoor education
15. Correspond for specific information and contact outside agencies
16. Plan health fairs and exhibits
17. Make models
18. Participate in panel discussions
19. Play records to demonstrate
20. Keep records (height and weight)
21. Plan a balanced menu—prepare and serve
22. Analyze data
23. Play games (educational)
24. Prepare bulletin boards
25. Collection of materials
26. Physical education competition (races)
27. Tutor other pupils
28. Puppet shows
29. Songs
30. Poetry

Students may also participate by teaching other students. "Studies of children teaching other children show that the child who teaches learns far more rapidly than the child who is taught. Also we need to help children think of themselves as lifelong students—to understand that their schooling is not finished when they leave the classroom."* The school nurse can be the effective leader, a resource person assisting the teacher along with the participating child and parent in health education.

---

*From Schaefer, Earl S.: A life-time, life-space perspective, Today's Education, p. 30, 1973.

Teaching methods

An effective method of dealing with the knowledge explosion of today was developed in 1967 by the School Health Education Study directed by Elena M. Sliepcevich.[1] This method identifies problems and converts them into instructional needs. A conceptual framework is expressed in three key concepts: (1) growing and developing, (2) interacting, and (3) decision making. The principles behind the conceptual approach are (1) the concept reveals a thought; the learner conceptualizes the relationship rather than memorizes isolated facts; and (2) the content is part of the process of learning. Having knowledge and facts are not sufficient to cope with the complexity of our problems. The conceptual approach offers a potential for imposing order on the variable environment.

California is one of the few states to develop the conceptual approach to health instruction; the *Framework for Health Instruction in California Public Schools, Twelfth Grade,*[2] was adopted by the California State Board of Education. This material is not a course of study but is used as a guide for local curriculum development. It is one of the few guides that includes concepts at grade levels—objectives and content suggestion. The ten areas of content are consumer health, mental-emotional health; drug use and misuse; family health; oral health, vision, and hearing; nutrition; exercise, rest, and posture; diseases and disorders; environmental health hazards; and community health resources.

A method that focuses on the learner's involvement in educating himself was described in a presentation, "The Nurse as a Health Educator," by Mary Louise Wilson[3] of the University of Utah School of Nursing. She explained a threefold nature of teaching, which is shown graphically in Fig. 6-2.

1. Preassessment
2. Learning activity

STUDENT	TEACHER
a. Perceive	Show
b. Think	Discuss
c. Try	Apply

3. Evaluation

The Cone of Learning Experiences shows that one learns by experience—the more real, the more permanent the learning (Fig. 6-3). Another method of learning is through brainstorming, which is centered on the principle of deferred judgment. This method may be combined with planned instruction that is particularly helpful for parent education.

The "Report of Parent Education and Special Project Activities" section of *Redirection of School Nursing Services* is an excellent source of information regard-

---

[1]Sliepcevich, Elena: Health education: a conceptual approach to curriculum design. Grades kindergarten through twelve, St. Paul, Minn., 1967, 3M Education Press.

[2]Hill, Patricia J., Fodor, John T., Gmur, Ben C., and Sutton, Wilfred C.: Framework for health instruction in California public schools, kindergarten through twelfth grade, Sacramento, Calif., 1970, California State Education Department.

[3]Wilson, Mary Louise: The nurse as a health educator, Proceedings of workshop for school nurses, Idaho State University, Department of Nursing, Pocatello, Idaho, 1970.

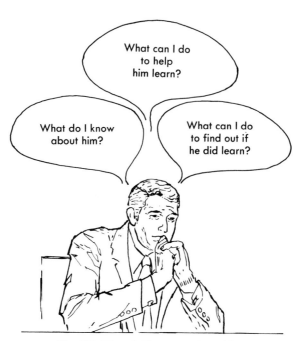

Fig. 6-2. Threefold nature of teaching.

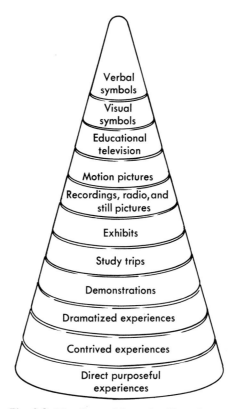

Fig. 6-3. The Cone of Learning Experiences.

ing parent participation. Parent education and child education activity was reported by giving reason for meeting, objectives, preparation, program, follow-up, and evaluation.[4] It may be helpful to suggest some of the topics for parent education:

1. Low-cost meal planning
2. Home economy and family life
3. Preparation for school
4. The importance of good dental health
5. Emotional and social development of the child
6. Divorce—its effects on children
7. Raising children in a large city
8. Teaching sex education to children
9. Weight of kindergarten children
10. Parent management of special problems
11. Immunizations
12. Persons to contact for special problems
13. Growth and development of 5-year-old children
14. These are your children
15. Parent health
16. Care of eyes
17. What to expect of your child entering the first grade
18. Human development
19. Discussion on drug abuse
20. Description of dental program

One can judge from this list that the needs of parents were considered important. Plans were made to satisfy the needs either by having a resource specialist, the school nurse, to answer questions and by using films and other resource material to participate in discussion.

In this same study some of the topics that nurses reported for groups of children and, in some cases, children and parents were as follows:

1. Nutritional needs of children
2. Dental examination
3. Keep a smile for the future
4. Good health habits
5. Animal nutrition study
6. Sleep and rest
7. Toothbrushing
8. Study of the lungs
9. Breakfast project
10. Health fair
11. Dental care
12. Care of hair
    a. Anatomy and growth of hair

---

[4]Bryan, Doris S., and Cook, Thelma T.: Redirection of school nursing services in culturally deprived neighborhoods, Final Report, Oakland, Calif., 1970, Oakland Public Schools.

b. Washing, drying, and styling
13. Skin care
14. Family life education
15. Communicable disease including venereal disease
16. Drug abuse
17. Care of nails
18. Diet and you
19. Nutrition: "Your food—choice or chance"

The educational opportunity for group teaching was planned and used effectively for the above topics of discussion. For health education one has to think of the possible methods and sources to help motivate both parents and children, such as follows:

1. Audiovisual aids
   a. Films
   b. Filmstrips
   c. Slides and tape
2. Textbooks—resource book
3. Professional library books available in the nurse's office
4. Pamphlets
5. Posters
6. Role playing
7. Ideas for activities in the classroom
   a. Bulletin boards and displays
   b. Drawings
   c. Discussions
   d. Dramatization
   e. Demonstrations
8. Excursions
9. Scrapbook
10. Speakers—students teaching students
11. Surveys

The task of changing attitudes and behavior in students to gain healthful living is a problem of coordinated effort of the home, school, and the community. A singular device that has been used to motivate students to change behavior is that of tape recordings. To know the world, one should have the opportunity to experience it, yet this is increasingly more difficult with the growing complexity of life.[5] Tape recordings of an individual telling his experiences can offer a substitute experience and assist students in conceptualizing their world. With careful selection of subjects, an individual telling his story stimulates interest, and it can be examined and communicated.

So it is with these various methods of approach to learning that the school nurse develops a sound health instructional program. The nurse's avenues of approach are with parents, teachers, and with the students themselves. Of course school health

[5]Hubbard, Nancy G.: Motivation for health learning: taped "live experience," J. Sch. Health 42:548, 1972.

instruction is only part of the total health education of students. They are influenced by experiences gained at home, the communication media, and in the community. However, there is an interrelatedness of health concepts that could be covered in various subjects such as social studies, science, physical education, and home economics. How health is stressed in the curriculum could very well depend on the school nurse to implement the health teaching and coordinate health materials.

HEALTH PROTOCOLS

Studies indicate that the written word is not the most effective method of instruction, but few schools can resist preparing health education materials for parents, teachers, and the nurses themselves. Health newsletters and bulletins are prevalent in most school health programs.

The following health protocols are examples of written information used by the nurse to assist parent and school personnel in understanding and coping with pupils with special problems: vision and hearing conservation—the care of the eyes; health classes on care of the ears; pupils with diabetes; considerations for students with convulsive disorders; a hearing health program for the parents; home eye tests for children age 1 to 7; and screening the educationally handicapped child.

FOR TEACHERS AND NURSES
Vision and hearing conservation—the care of the eyes*

INTERMEDIATE GRADES

Preparing children for vision screening. Before the vision screening program is initiated, motivation and preparation are needed. This protocol is one approach that may be used.

Materials needed. The following materials are needed: light meter, model of human eye, eye chart, and Snellen eye chart.

I. Discuss importance of the eye
   A. In animals, birds, and fish
      1. Hippopotamus—eyes are on top of its head to permit the hippopotamus to watch for danger while keeping most of its huge body submerged in water.
      2. Hawk—living animals are captured and killed instantly for food. A hawk can see a fast-moving animal at a great distance with its sharp eyesight.
   B. In human beings
      1. Have children list the number of ways in which the eye is important to man.
II. Motivation—create interest by use of game involving all the children in the class to initiate this study.
   A. Name the Objects—have fifteen or twenty small, covered objects on table. Explain to the children that the objects will be uncovered for them to ob-

---

*Adapted from Judy, Elizabeth: Group IV vision and hearing conservation, Proceedings of workshop for school nurses, Idaho State University, Department of Nursing, Pocatello, Idaho, 1970.

serve for 15 seconds. The objects should then be recovered and the children asked to list on paper as many of the objects as possible.

III. Reasons for vision screening
    A. Question, "Why do we do the vision screening test each year?"
    B. Answer, "Eyes change from year to year, and more rapidly during childhood than in later life."

IV. Discuss natural protection of eye
    A. Position of eye in the skull (Use eye model. Let children take the model apart, examine it, and put the eye model back together.)
        1. Set in for protection
    B. Eyelids
        1. Protect surface of eyes
            a. Quick blinking protects eye from flying objects, insects, blows, etc.
    C. Eyebrows and eyelashes
        1. Afford protection
            a. Raise question, "How do our eyebrows and eyelashes protect our eyes?"
    D. Tear glands
        1. Moisten and protect surface of eye

V. Importance of eyes—why they should have every advantage.
    A. We get just one pair of eyes in a lifetime. Let's take care of them.
    B. We use our eyes for reading, study, work, and play.
    C. "Who can mention other ways in which we use our eyes?"
        1. Earning our living as adults
        2. Enjoying beautiful scenery
        3. Recreation, games, sports, etc.
        4. Reading directions on how to cook, build model planes, etc.

FOR TEACHERS AND NURSES
Health classes on care of the ears*

INTERMEDIATE GRADES

Explain the anatomy and functions of the different parts of the ear, using the ear model and audiometer chart.

Materials needed

1. Ear model
2. Audiometer chart (Beltone, Maico, etc.)
3. Wash cloth, soap, towel, small basin with water
4. Sharp objects (bobby pin, pencil, etc.)
5. Bean, button, or other small object
6. Paraffin to represent earwax
7. Balloon to represent eardrum

---

*Adapted from Judy, Elizabeth: Group IV vision and hearing conservation, Proceedings of workshop for school nurses, Idaho State University, Department of Nursing, Pocatello, Idaho, 1970.

Demonstration

I. How to cleanse the ear correctly
   A. With a wash cloth, soap, towel, and small basin of water, show class how to wash the ear correctly by using ear model.
   B. Discuss with the class the importance of clean ears.
II. Dangers of hard blows to the head
   A. Blow up a balloon to simulate the eardrum and have a child break the balloon.
   B. Have the class compare the similarity of the balloon to what happens to the eardrum:
      1. When we fall
      2. By the impact of water when diving
      3. By loud blasts or explosions
III. Dangers of sharp objects
   A. Using an inflated balloon to simulate eardrum, have a child break balloon with a sharp instrument (bobby pin, pencil, etc.).
   B. Have the class compare the similarity of the breaking of the balloon to what happens when eardrum is punctured with a sharp instrument.
IV. Dangers of a foreign object in the ear
   A. Using an ear model, place a bean, button, or other small object in outer ear and show how it can be worked toward the eardrum.

Do not put anything smaller than your elbow into your ear!

Ear care. Have the class discuss, after you have demonstrated to them the danger of trying to remove a foreign body yourself, the need for medical attention.

Impairment of hearing due to excessive wax. Place a small amount of paraffin into ear model. Have the group discuss the protective function of earwax and how impaired hearing can result from excessive wax.

FOR SCHOOL PERSONNEL—TEACHERS WITH DIABETIC STUDENTS
Pupils with diabetes*

It is important that school personnel recognize the signs of an insulin reaction of a child with diabetes.

Signs of an insulin reaction. The first signs of an insulin reaction are usually paleness, sweating, and trembling or shakiness. The child may exhibit one or all of these signs at once or may only show one of them for several minutes. It is important to realize that there is no usual order in the occurrence of these signs even in the same individual at different times.

The child may complain of a headache, feeling faint or weak, dizzy, hungry, nauseated, or may "see double." His coordination may show such changes as inability to do such simple things as turn a page, write, or speak clearly. These complaints, likewise, do not occur in a definite order. Sometimes headache may be the only complaint for some time, or the child may complain first of nausea.

*Developed by the Nursing Services Department, Oakland Public Schools, Oakland, Calif.

Most diabetic children are quickly aware of the onset of an insulin reaction and may tell the teacher, "Something is wrong—I don't feel good" instead of stating exactly what is wrong. This is because in an insulin reaction it is not uncommon to have mental and physical coordination affected at the onset, and clear thinking is impossible. Unconsciousness or coma occasionally occurs before any other sign is noted.

If a diabetic child has any of the above complaints or signs, sugar or fruit juice should be given if the child, himself, does not have any. Usually diabetic children are taught very early to always have a few lumps of sugar or a candy bar with them.

If a diabetic child has a reaction in school, even if sugar or juice is taken and he apparently is all right in a few minutes, the parent should be contacted and the child taken home by the parent or a member of the school staff.

Suggestions to teachers. When you first know of any diabetic child in your classroom, you should talk over the situation with his parents and with him and make every effort to establish confidence and understanding of his problem. Children, especially during adolescence, may be difficult to "stabilize" from the standpoint of adjusting the amount of insulin to activity and rapid development; and it is not unusual for them to have quite a few insulin reactions from time to time during this period of development.

Find out from the child and his parent if he carries sugar or a candy bar. Likewise, find out if the child has any usual first signs or complaints with an insulin reaction.

It is a good idea to have a few lumps of sugar or a candy bar in your desk in case the child forgets to bring his.

FOR SCHOOL PERSONNEL—TEACHERS WITH STUDENTS WITH CONVULSIVE DISORDERS
Considerations for students with convulsive disorders*

Identification and reporting of cases. When the school first learns that a child has a convulsive disorder such as epilepsy from a past health record, health history, or the occurrence of an attack, it is the responsibility of the nurse to determine whether or not the student is receiving medical supervision and to learn the medical recommendations for the student's school program.

A report of all cases and the medical recommendations for each should be submitted to the principal and counselor or classroom teacher.

Information about convulsive disorders. Heredity, disturbances of prenatal environment, birth injuries, infections and accidents in early life, allergy, and malnutrition are *all* causes of convulsive disorders in children.

Progress in medical treatment now enables us to regard patients with controlled epilepsy as normal human beings, handicapped only temporarily when convulsive episodes occur. Today most patients can have their illness properly diagnosed and so well controlled by medication that their seizures are mild and infrequent. It is seldom that spells in children are so frequent or severe that nonattendance at school

---

*Developed by the Nursing Services Department, Oakland Public Schools, Oakland, Calif.

is warranted; and when suspension from school is approved, it is usually only a temporary arrangement.

Attending school and being happily occupied with normal activities usually lessens social tension that precipitates seizures. It is unwise to overprotect the child by keeping him segregated between attacks. Physical activity, regular or modified, is usually encouraged. There is often a relationship between inactivity and seizures; a constant flutter before the eyes as on television may precipitate attacks.

Intellectually the epileptic child is not greatly dissimilar to the nonepileptic child. If given suitable opportunity, the epileptic child has the same ability to learn as has a child who is physically normal.

The two most common types of seizures are grand mal and petit mal.

Grand mal In this type of seizure the patient loses consciousness, his muscles tighten, and he falls. He may cry out or groan, although he does not remember pain. Saliva appears on his lips. His face may be first dusky and then pale. He twitches violently for a minute or so—it seems much longer to the worried bystander. Usually in a few minutes he lies relaxed. The patient is not uncomfortable during a seizure; he is unconscious of it.

Petit mal The seizures are much more frequent but are often overlooked because they last only a few seconds. The patient may stare vacantly, blink his eyes, and appear slightly confused.

If children are forewarned of the possibility of a seizure occurring and informed about the disease, when they witness a seizure in the presence of a calm teacher, their usual reaction is sympathy mixed with wholesome curiosity, rather than terror and panic.

Procedures to follow when a seizure occurs in school. The child should be trained to be accompanied, preferably by understanding friends, at all times.

Petit mal seizure requires little attention except to pick up anything the child may drop without objecting to the incident. The teacher should realize that the student may have missed a short portion of classroom discussion.

If a child should have a *grand mal or convulsive seizure,* follow these directions:

1. Ease student to the floor and loosen collar. Do not try to restrain the jerking.
2. Turn head to one side for easy release of saliva and place some padding under his head for comfort.
3. Move away furniture and hard objects that he might strike while jerking.
4. It is *not* necessary to put something between his teeth.
5. Assign someone to watch the patient until jerking stops. The other members of the class should continue with class instruction as in any other medical emergency. (Situations vary.)
6. After jerking has ceased, a small child can be carried to a restroom until ready to resume activity, and a large child allowed to lie until able to walk there.
7. Notify parent. When attack is over, student may continue with his school schedule unless parent or student requests otherwise. If it is a known epileptic case, it is not usually necessary to call a doctor immediately.
8. No accident report is necessary for an uncomplicated seizure; a report is necessary only when the child may have received some physical injury as from a fall.

FOR PARENTS AND SCHOOL PERSONNEL
A hearing health program for the parents*

Parents may not know that their child does not hear well. Although he may hear when he is standing nearby or seated at the table, he should hear the same loudness many feet away or even upstairs. A child has a margin of hearing that may gradually lessen until the hearing loss is noticeable. Then it may be too late. It is wise to give periodic tests and to care for small hearing losses when discovered to prevent them from becoming greater and permanent.

The following simple rules are offered as a guide to good hearing health:

1. *Earaches* mean "The child is sick." Find out why he is sick. A bad earache is very dangerous. Children who do not get prompt medical attention may have some permanent hearing loss later.

2. A *running ear* is dangerous to the child's life and health. Never fail to call on the ear doctor for help. A running ear may cause much destruction of the hearing.

3. *Lancing the ear* does not destroy the hearing. It saves the drum membrane from a rupture that may leave a hole or scar.

4. *Frequent colds and sniffles* often affect the hearing. Keep the child's health at his best. If the child does have a cold, treat the cold at once. Do not let it "drag on." Find out what causes frequent colds.

5. *If one or both ears "close up"* during a cold, go to the doctor at once.

6. *Diseased adenoids and tonsils* may aggravate colds and ear troubles. They may cause middle ear abscesses or close the opening between the ear and throat, which may result in a hearing loss.

7. *Mouth breathing* usually, but not always, indicates adenoids or other nasal obstructions. Any unhealthy condition of the nose and throat may affect the hearing.

8. *Hearing losses* may occur so gradually that no one knows about them. Light but long-standing inflammations of the sinuses or nasal passages may stealthily attack the hearing. It is said that an acute attack, when treated, offers greater chance of recovery of normal hearing than the gradual assault on the ear by light infections such as catarrh, which may result in a gradual irreversible loss of hearing.

9. *Contagious diseases,* such as scarlet fever, measles, diphtheria, mumps, and whooping cough, give ear troubles to many children, especially the young. Avoid exposure of your child and take advantage of inoculations.

   CAUTION: Watch the child's ears for aches and discharge *during* and *after* the disease. Ask the doctor to watch too. Quickly obtain treatment if trouble occurs. Much permanent loss can be prevented through prompt action.

10. *Wax or objects* in children's ears may cause a hearing loss. If you cannot remove it with a damp cloth over the end of your finger, only the doctor should remove it. Wax may be packed in the ear so hard that repeated treatments may be required for its removal. Some children must go to doctors occasionally for wax removal.

---

*Developed by the Nursing Services Department, Oakland Public Schools, Oakland, Calif.

11. *Defective teeth* and other mouth infections may affect the hearing. Consult the dentist.

12. *Undernourishment* leaves the body susceptible to infections and ear troubles. consult the doctor about suitable foods for your child.

13. *Progressive deafness* of the inherited type may begin early in childhood. Although restoration may be impossible, much can be done to alleviate that condition and help the child. Lip reading skills should be acquired early.

14. *Some "don'ts" for good hearing health:*

    a. Don't let a child get water in his ear if there is a hole in the drum membrane.

    b. Don't let a child swim in any but controlled pools to prevent ear infection.

    c. Don't let a child subject to ear troubles swim except with a doctor's permission. Diving and crawl stroke should be prohibited. Breaststroke permits the head to be kept above water.

    d. Avoid colds as much as possible in the child with ear trouble and treat promptly if he should get one. Don't let him wet his hair for combing. Make him wear a hat in cold weather.

    e. Don't wash the ear canal with soap. Use a damp cloth. Soap irritates the canal, and the child might scratch the ear with a soiled finger.

    f. Don't let children box or shout into each other's ears.

    g. Don't use homemade or over-the-counter remedies for an earache. Get the doctor's advice. You may use the most undesirable remedy.

    h. Don't let them put objects or "poke" into the ears.

    i. Don't think a child is stubborn when he doesn't answer habitually. Investigate his hearing.

    j. Don't forget that hearing varies from time to time under different conditions.

    k. Don't think a child will "outgrow" his hearing loss. The loss may remain the same, but his attention could improve. The hearing of many children gets worse.

    l. Don't let a child blow his nose loudly or with one or both nostrils partly closed, especially during a cold. It is advisable to lean slightly forward when blowing the nose. Don't blow the nose while lying on the back. Infectious materials are easily forced into the middle ear.

    m. Don't delay having the ears tested if you suspect a hearing loss. When the loss is obvious, it may be too late to help the child.

    n. Don't forget that most defects of hearing are preventable! Many adults trace their ear troubles back to childhood days!

It is good sense to take care of the ears.

FOR PARENTS
Home eye tests for children age 1 to 7*

There are about one million children in this country who have faulty vision in one eye. If this condition is found early enough, it is possible to save the vision in the affected eye. Two simple home vision tests for children in this age group are available to you.

Instructions for the "E" test (age 1 to 7) (Fig. 6-4)

1. Show the enclosed "E" chart to your child and teach him how to indicate the direction of the "E" with his hand and fingers.
2. When he can do that, patch one eye, "like Captain Hook," and have him sit 10 feet from you.
3. Hold the "E" chart in front of you at waist level, making sure the chart is well illuminated.
4. Begin at the top of the "E" chart and point to the various "E" symbols with your finger. Ask your child to indicate the direction of the "E" by pointing his fingers in the right direction.
5. Change the patch over to the other eye and repeat the test.
6. Most children in this age group will see the second smallest line.

Instructions for the candy bead test (age 2 to 4)

1. Show the capsule containing the tiny candy beads to your child and let him taste a few of them.
2. Place a white towel on the floor and put three of the candy beads on the towel about a foot apart from each other.
3. Allow your child to pick them up using both eyes.
4. Ask your child to pick them up with one eye open while the other eye is covered with the patch. Then test the other eye.
5. He should be able to see the beads with each eye from the standing position.

*Adapted from Judy, Elizabeth: Group IV vision and hearing conservation, Proceedings of workshop for school nurses, Idaho State University, Department of Nursing, Pocatello, Idaho, 1970.

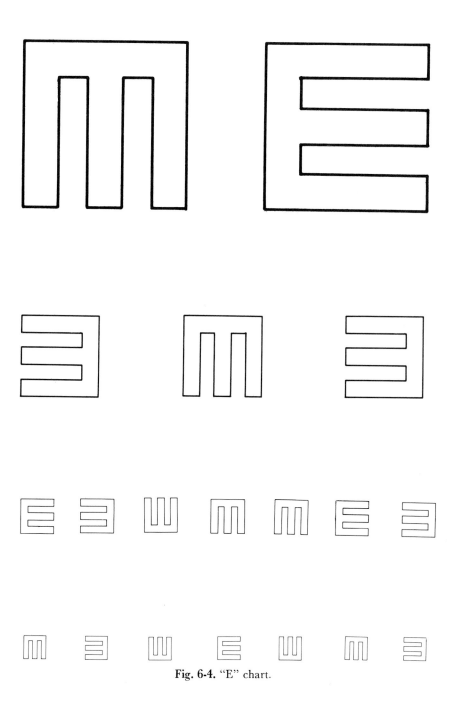

Fig. 6-4. "E" chart.

Screening the educationally handicapped child*

How to identify an educationally handicapped child. Although most of these symptoms may be observed in normal children, the educationally handicapped appear to have an unusually high incidence of the difficulties in the following outline.

I. Prenatal and birth history
   A. Mother had history of complicated pregnancies
   B. Child born prematurely or after prolonged pregnancy
   C. Delivery precipitate or prolonged
   D. Breech, transverse, or footling presentation
   E. Unusual amount of drug or anesthetics
   F. Anoxia
   G. Blood transfusions

II. Health history
   A. Convulsions
   B. Excessively high fevers
   C. Loss of consciousness (due to head injury, illness, unexplained)
   D. Unusual feeding pattern (excessive colic, projectile vomiting, etc.)
   E. Hyper- or hypoactive (infancy, preschool, school)
   F. Physical abnormalities (abnormal gait, etc.)
   G. Major illnesses or accidents, accident proneness
   H. Emotional problems

III. Developmental history
   A. Delayed speech or unusual articulation
   B. Delay in sitting, standing, walking, etc.
   C. Late toilet training, prolonged enuresis
   D. Poor large or small muscle coordination

IV. Screening observation data
   A. Poor auditory acuity and discrimination
   B. Poor visual acuity and discrimination
   C. Poor eye-muscle balance and control
   D. Poor directionality and/or confused laterality
   E. Significant problems identified on preschool physical
   F. Medical information currently available

No one finding is significant by itself. Each must be interpreted in light of all available information.

---

*Adapted from Cantrell, Mary: Group VII school nurses' role in special education, Proceedings of workshop for school nurses, Idaho State University, Department of Nursing, Pocatello, Idaho, 1970.

SUMMARY MODEL
Student health and safety convention*

The health convention is an enjoyable and excellent means of culminating health education activities for all levels in education: elementary, intermediate, secondary, and college. Below is an example of a successful health convention in the Mount Diablo School District, Concord, California.

STUDENT ADVANTAGES
1. Sharing of information
2. Motivation to learn more about health
3. Reward for work done in health and safety councils
4. Acquiring new ideas
5. Experience in group dynamics
6. Experience as an individual representing a group with the dual responsibility to group and to convention
7. Provides an opportunity for children to gain experience in verbal communication as leaders, recorders, and as members of a group
8. Provides experience in speaking before large groups

STAFF ADVANTAGES
1. Added opportunity for group of school staff in gaining new concepts in teaching health

COMMUNITY ADVANTAGES
1. It gives key people in health fields the opportunity to become familiar with health programs in the schools.
2. It gives them an opportunity to be a participant observer with school-age children.
3. Provides an opportunity for children of the Mt. Diablo Unified School District to gain firsthand information with community resources in health and safety and how to utilize them through personal contact.

FUTURE PLANNING
1. Plans for the health and safety convention should be initiated early in the school year, appointing general chairman and subcommittee chairman from school staff.
2. This project should be endorsed by the school district for full cooperation and support.
3. The date, place, and theme of convention placed on school calendar early in fall of school year.
4. Principals should be informed of availability of substitutes for teacher sponsors.
5. Nursing staff should be encouraged to fully participate in this program.
6. Jane Krigin should be assigned as student health convention adviser.

*This is the fourteenth year of this activity. Parents, pupils, teachers, and the community demand its continuance.

7. The new committee should carefully consider previous convention evaluations and recommendations.
8. Convention summary should be prepared for use by the following year's planning committee members.

The following account of the convention was reported in "Health Headlines," a newsletter of the Contra Costa County Health Department, Martinez, California:

"How do the foods we eat affect our health?" "How can we make our environment cleaner and healthier?" "What courses of action might we take in the face of certain disaster conditions?"

These and other thought-provoking questions were handled in adult fashion by an inspired group of elementary school youngsters in the Annual School Health and Safety Convention, held at the Clayton Valley School May 16th. This year's all day program, comprised of 4th, 5th and 6th grade representatives of eight schools in the Mt. Diablo District, bore the theme "Health Freedoms," signifying the open door to attaining long range health objectives. In a refreshing display of talent, originality and good old hard work, the students went about to prove quite conclusively that health and safety consciousness can be effectively stimulated at the younger age levels.

The morning half of the program was ushered in by a warm welcome from Clayton Valley Principal, Mr. Lloyd Gass. After a musical interlude by the school glee club, Mr. Gass introduced a talented 6th grade master of ceremonies who called upon the participating schools, one at a time, to tell their respective accomplishments in the field of health. Each school reported on a specific topic (as nutrition, safety, sanitation, civil defense, physical fitness, dental health, health attitudes and immunization). A life-sized T.V. screen, made by the Glenbrook School woodshop, served as the stage setting, and each school, identified by "channel" number, gave its presentation in the form of a skit, recitation, or poetry. The morning concluded with a play about the human body performed by the Dramatic Club of Clayton Valley School.

At noon the conventioners enjoyed a well-balanced lunch (the menu was designed by students and selected on a competitive basis for best food value). Mealtime entertainment was provided by capable musical and dancing performers. Next the group was conducted through the Youth Center where a number of health and safety displays made by students were exhibited. These included puppet shows, posters, project books, clay models of organs of the body, and similar creations.

During the afternoon session eight separate round-table discussions on different health topics took place. These were attended by elected delegates from the different schools, their teen age advisor, an adult observer and a qualified resource person, as a health department sanitarian, county safety officer, or assistant health officer. Here the students had the opportunity to discuss a few of the challenging personal and community health problems under capable guidance by an expert in the particular field. The discussion followed the principles of free expression, teamwork, and good leadership, and one could well envision tomorrow's community leaders in the making. The administrator and health consultant of the Clayton Valley School are to be commended on their splendid planning and promotional activities which involved so many community resources.

The School Health and Safety Council got its start in the Clayton Valley School six years ago under the auspices of the school health consultant, Mrs. Jane Krigin. She had observed a minimum of organized interest in health and safety activities in the schools to which she had been assigned as nurse. As a method to promote group action, she proposed the Student Health and Safety Council, which received strong administrative endorsement. Her plan called for 4th through

6th graders, two elected from each classroom, to meet weekly or whenever a health emergency should arise, and convey thoughts gleaned from the meetings back to the classroom for discussion. Also included in her scheme were annual health assemblies, forerunners of the present health conventions. After working out a few changes in format, the proposed council became a reality, operating in high gear almost from the start.

Agenda for council meetings includes suggestions from students, parents or faculty, field trips to health and safety agencies (as the water treatment plant), special projects, discussions on ways to promote healthful activities, and use of outside resources. The students might invite the police department for a talk on bicycle licensing and safety; the cafeteria supervisor to discuss meal planning; or the dental society to help plan posters. They have learned how to use effectively such devices as cheers, animal experiments, films, newsletters and demonstrations of healthful techniques.

The gathering together of delegates of the several student health councils at a convention is a new activity within the school. It demonstrates that health awareness is possible at all age levels, even in the kindergarten. Each year the Health and Safety Councils of other schools have asked to participate in the convention. The council is a two-way street: the students learn to develop health attitudes, and the school staff is assisted in developing health curriculum units and projects.

The sponsors of the Clayton Valley program have, in addition, undertaken the ambitious task of involving adults of the community in health and safety problems of the school, emphasizing the need for the coordinated approach to community health matters. The possibilities of establishing such adult health councils and coordinating their efforts with those of the School Health and Safety group should be further exploited.

Still to be achieved, and not too far in the future, we hope, is the realization of one of the long range goals of the council, the Health Museum. Therein would lie the concrete evidence of measurable accomplishment, and the symbol of high scholastic achievement in health in our county's schools.

7

SCHOOL AND COMMUNITY LIAISON

In most school districts the school nurse has more opportunity than other school personnel to be the liaison person between school and community resources, including parents, official and voluntary health agencies, and the medical and dental communities.

The nurse must keep abreast with current programs available to children and youth and can often be instrumental in obtaining new resources for health and welfare needs in the community. In her routine activities of referrals for defects and through contacts with parents, teachers, community agencies, or other school specialists, the nurse must be able to recognize the problem and interpret it to others. These important functions of school nurses are among the reasons why the school nurse must acquire the knowledges and skills of community health nursing in her preparation.

COMMUNICATION

Nurses need to know how to listen, about interaction among people, and about individual and group counseling techniques. It is often difficult for professional persons to learn to listen because they are accustomed to directing or supervising others. Listening combined with a respect for others can result in decisions promoting advantageous change for both the school and the community.

Listening. The school nurse is often the only person who knows the reasons for problems that contribute to a child's learning or behavioral difficulties. It may be that the "nurse is the only one who has listened to a child long enough to find out how he lives and/or visited his home. The nurse knows how he feels about himself, his life at home, his life at school, including how he feels about his teacher and how he perceives the teacher feels about him."* Home visiting has long been the role of the school nurse; it is a very important activity for gathering facts, knowing the needs that exist, and taking time for listening to people relate their problems; home visits also help the nurse formulate solutions to the problems found. The school nurse is the liaison between the home and the school and is needed for interpreting the health-related findings.

Respect for others. The human right to differ is becoming more and more ap-

---

*From Outman, Margaret H.: The school nurse and community agencies, Workshop Proceedings for School Nurses, fourth general session, Idaho State University, Pocatello, Idaho, 1970.

130

parent in this changing world. Doctors and nurses again have difficulty in this area where for so many years they have expected their opinions and directives to be followed without question. It must be remembered that other people's values, actions, and priorities may be just as appropriate and right, or perhaps more so than the time-honored ways of doing things.

It is important for nurses to leave the door open for better communication and understanding. This attitude can be put into practice through the use of such statements as "that is a good idea but let's see if there are some other points of view," or "have you ever thought of this?" This process may be more time consuming in either individual or group counseling, but learning various points of view and making a group decision usually result in a more appropriate, meaningful solution.

If the school nurse can interact with parents, teachers, and students, the school soon becomes family centered. Here again, attitudes are important. Many parents are afraid of teachers and fear coming to school. Likewise, there are teachers who fear communicating with parents. In order to overcome these feelings, some schools have organized parent study groups. These groups choose a topic of mutual interest pertaining to school activities and study it in depth. Study groups were also mentioned in Chapter 6.

Decisions. It is only natural to hope to make correct decisions and assessments of situations at all times but mere humans cannot always be right. A judgment made in haste and under stress has more chances of being inaccurate. So if at all possible, take a second look at a situation when emotions are not so strong.

Often if humor can be brought into the situation in dealing with others, or if a smile or a sincere compliment can be given, the situation will be put back into perspective, both for nurse as well as others. These ideas are worth trying when working with other people.

There is no better way of understanding personal views than to reduce them to the spoken or written word, However, before speaking or writing so that others can get the intended meaning—*think*. A clearly written or spoken statement is an invaluable aid in communication and in effective decision making.

Change. School nurses should never underestimate their fellow workers in the promotion of mental, physical, and social health of pupils. A few of their co-workers include pupil personnel workers, speech therapists, food service personnel, custodial services, instructional supervisors, and the librarians.

School curriculums often remain in a stable position by adhering to certain principles. It is the pressure from parents and community personnel that eventually effects change. New approaches and research studies are of real value for a progressive school district to answer the needs on a local level. Working together requires the art of communication. It was the novelist Joseph Conrad who once remarked, "Give me the right word and accent and I will move the world."

COMMUNITY COOPERATION

School nurses in transition are finding themselves involved in community planning projects. As suburbia develops, the nurse is able to contribute where plans will affect the lives of children. The community leaders need the benefit of the school nurse when planning recreation centers, clinics, service centers, drug programs, housing projects, mental health services, and job placement programs. What makes nurses valuable members of the planning team is that they are knowledgeable of the community resources and can suggest sources of help needed.

Parents and students often need to be told about and encouraged to accept and use health services where they are available. This is a matter of education. It is also the role of the nurse to help doctors and dentists to be aware of the services that the school nurse offers the community, the school, the home, and to medical and dental practice. It is important in respect to the community to interpret the advances in school nursing. More than ever before the professions are operating as *health teams*. "We have a responsibility to the American people to collaborate in studying, experimenting and working toward the development of the most effective possible systems of providing health care."* This gives school nurses the responsibility of interpreting their role of and deciding whether their potential is being used effectively for the school and the community. The modern technical advances to improve health care will never replace the empathetic, knowledgeable nurse. It has been said, "I have an electric toothbrush. I see my dentist two times a year. But I see my electrician three times a week." School nurses will adapt these new technological advances so that their personal services may be used to the best advantage.

Community projects are often introduced at school when student participation is required. Children are reminded of vaccination time for pet animals to prevent rabies, bicycle safety—license program, and kite-flying safety. Many schools participate in programs of safety patrols that guide students to and from school, thus informing students of their responsibilities early in life.

Voluntary health agencies. Voluntary health agencies are often excellent resources for the schools. Many agencies employ trained public health educators who can provide expert service as consultants and who can give information concerning health media resources and funds for special projects and programs. Again, the nurse must interpret needs and the contribution of school health services to these groups. All community health agencies need an interpretation of the total structure of the school administration and its commitment to education, since many agencies believe schoolchildren and their parents are captive audiences for their particular health message.

Parent advisory groups. The school may benefit by a parent advisory committee such as an adult health council. Pupil health councils may also be effective in solving health problems and motivating students' learning. If parents and students can express their feelings, the school nurse is usually able to assist with the problem. "Some schools have sponsored health fairs where doctors and dentists participate with student groups. The response has been very gratifying where the professional personnel, parents, and pupils meet in solving their local health problems. Doctors become aware of the real needs as expressed by students and parents. Parents and students become informed of the professional viewpoint."† Perhaps doctors will consider

---

*From Wilbur, Dwight L.: Total manpower needs and resources—medicine and nursing, Nurs. Outlook **17**:32, 1969.

†From Krigin, Jane, and Gass, Lloyd: A student health and safety council at Clayton Valley School, J. Sch. Health **29**:67, 1959.

the health inventory more carefully and do more than communicate by an illegible note of "healthy child."

The health department. Cooperative efforts between the school and the health department are many. Examples of how cooperative policies may be written follow:

1. *Policies and procedures on tuberculosis control*

The school is expected to include the study of communicable disease in the health curriculum. Protective procedures and policies have been established for suspected and active cases for tuberculosis control. The eligibility for home instruction has been defined, and the procedure for contacts to infectious cases in school has been outlined. All of these procedures have to be reviewed cooperatively, including the positive tuberculin test cases found in school.

2. *Policies on interviewing students for venereal disease contacts*

The positive, instructive approach seems to be the effective way to investigate this ever-present problem. The lines of responsibility must be defined between the school and the health department.

BARRIERS TO LIAISON

A barrier to the team approach is the school nurse who is overly compulsive to do everything for the patient. At the other extreme is the nurse who lacks concern and who takes it for granted that the family will assume responsibility for care of the child. The effectiveness of the nurse in working together in the team is the nurse's ability to exercise professional judgment in assuming the responsibilities that belong to nursing and of respecting and understanding the roles of fellow team members.[1]

School nurses must recognize their own strengths and weaknesses, be firm in what they should do professionally on the job, and not be coaxed into assuming responsibilities that do not require nursing knowledge. The extent to which nurses perform in a highly professional manner in schools depends upon their own philosophies, goals, and commitments to nursing.

Since we assume school nurses usually work independently within the school and are the sole health resource within the school, they cannot work in a vacuum. They must develop with others a school nursing program to meet the needs of their particular school population. They work with the school team, as well as parents and community, to meet these needs. The nurse's function and responsibilities are not always the same and the barriers she must overcome are not always the same, but the importance of her role as a liaison to the community is a part of school nursing in transition.

SUMMARY MODEL

If school nursing services were placed on a pie graph with wedges assigned to various members of the health team, wedges would differ in size according to the nature of each pupil, his problem, the ability of the family to assume responsibility for care, and the availability of others to help. This pie would vary during the course of contact (Figs. 7-1 to 7-9).

[1]American Journal of Nursing, Co. Ed. Services Division: Changing patterns of nursing practice—new needs, new roles, 1971.

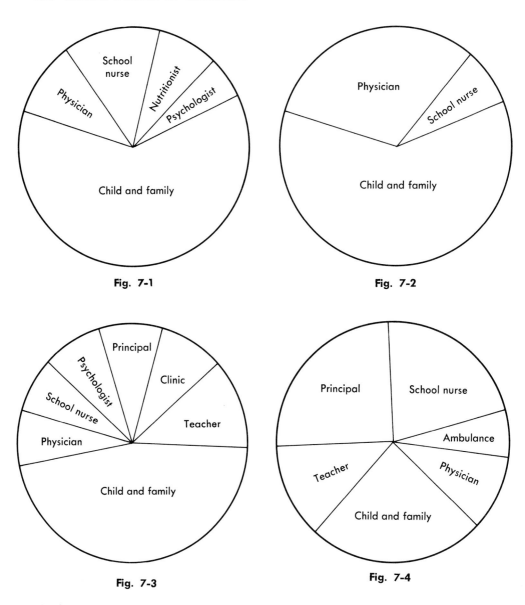

Fig. 7-1.

Fig. 7-2.

Fig. 7-3

Fig. 7-4

Fig. 7-1. Teen-ager under treatment for obesity. For successful treatment this team included the family, nutritionist, school nurse, and physician. Perhaps the school psychologist would also be involved.

Fig. 7-2. Adolescent under treatment for acne in a doctor's office. The school nurse implemented the treatment for this student, but the nurse has a minor part to play in treatment.

Fig. 7-3. Disturbed 10-year-old boy under treatment in mental health clinic. Several disciplines are represented here to assist this child.

Fig. 7-4. Major accident at school. The nurse and principal are taking a leading role in this problem.

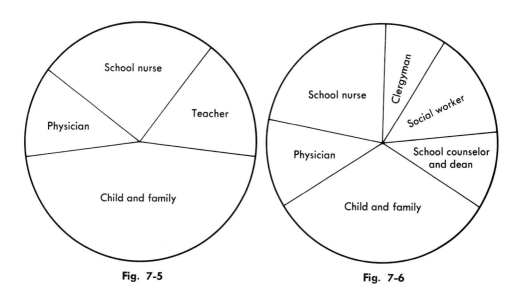

Fig. 7-5   **Fig. 7-6**

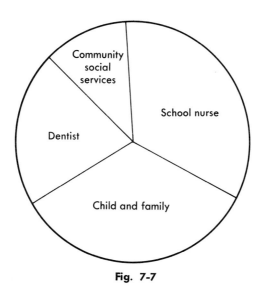

Fig. 7-7

Fig. 7-5. Child with brain tumor referred to nurse for eye test by teacher at school. An alert teacher and an informed nurse handled this problem.

Fig. 7-6. Pregnant teen-ager. Many disciplines were involved with this pupil.

Fig. 7-7. Mother seeking dental care for family. A conscientious mother and a nurse well informed of community resources were important in this case.

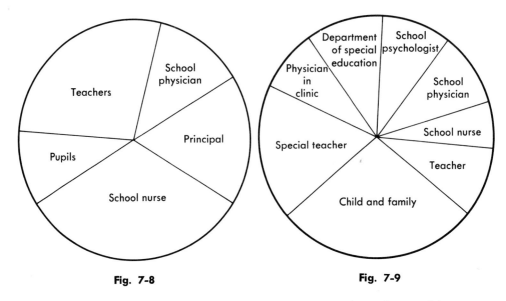

Fig. 7-8

Fig. 7-9

Fig. 7-8. Nurse planning in-service health education program. A steering or advisory committee ascertained needs, found appropriate resources, and worked out means of implementation.

Fig. 7-9. Mentally retarded child considered for placement in special program. Let us hope the child and his family are not overcome by the number of "experts" handling this case.

8

PROGRAM PLANNING AND EVALUATION

School nurses accomplish their goals by their ability to (1) envision needs, (2) plan for scheduled activities, and (3) adapt schedules for flexibility. These goals are best accomplished by planning toward definite objectives. The evaluative process includes planning sessions with the school administrator or other school personnel, the teacher, and the coordinator of health services. At these sessions policies, procedures, and objectives of the school health program can be evaluated and priorities for the program can be set. Guidelines for expectations will give direction for necessary improvement. Everyone wants children to become what they are capable of becoming. The cooperative effort is a shared responsibility and can be used as an effective tool for improvement. Changes happen by cooperative action of the school and the community personnel.

MEASURING OUTCOMES
Health services

It is difficult to measure the outcome of a school health program, but the method generally used in the process includes the following steps:
1. State the objectives.
2. List behavioral objectives to be considered in evaluation.
3. Select measuring devices.
4. Keep records of findings.
5. Interpret findings to improve the health program.

The evaluation of the health program would examine health services, health instruction, faculty and parent-community participation, counseling and guidance facilities, student health appraisal, and professional qualities of the school nurse. This is no easy task, but for too long students have returned facts that teachers have wanted to hear—yet, have school nurses changed behavior or applied health information in appropriate ways?

One deterrent in measuring outcomes is the budget. A relatively new screening device in health programs is the use of the phonocardioscan for heart-sound screening. This is usually only feasible in large health programs because of the cost, yet a justification for screening has been that this is one way to detect rheumatic and congenital heart conditions[1, 2] and to detect students whose parents assume their

---

[1]Eisner, Victor, and Oglesby, Allan: Health assessment of school children VII heart sound screening, J. Sch. Health **42:**270, 1972.
[2]Eisner, V., and Callan, L. C.: Dimensions of school health, Springfield, Ill., Charles C Thomas, Publisher. (In press.)

children have heart disease and make "heart cripples" of them through misunderstandings of physicians' findings. The budget and funding of an evaluative procedure are the crux of many good health programs.

Some areas such as dental examinations and treatment, cleanliness, posture, reports of changed behavior made by parents, and increase in percentage of physical defects remedied can be measured. Checklists and rating scales for health performances, personality inventories, and rating for school behavior and attitudes are available, but useful elementary health education devices are lacking.

The common measuring devices used for health services are observation, interviews, screening procedures, checklists, surveys, and analysis of records. A list or guide of what to look for is of value in health appraisals. School nurses usually assume the responsibility for screening procedures. Teachers may observe faulty eating habits, undue fatigue, failure to wash hands after using the toilet, and other performance encounters. The health appraisal and knowing the contributing factors of a learning disorder would certainly facilitate remediation.

Studies for early identification of characteristics that are related to future problems are of prime importance. A study reported by Lampe[3] showed a high correlation between the teacher's judgment and the prediction of nurses who used the interview technique. The contribution of interviews with students and with their parents, visits to their homes, and guidance counseling in helping students to accept and adjust positively to their limitations may provide a valuable means of appraising health problems.

Along with the health appraisal the school nurse keeps records, reports, and statistical information. The student's cumulative record on health progress may be revealing because of anecdotal accounts. Records of the measurement of physical performance tests help to indicate special health needs. Body mechanics and posture may be related to malnutrition, chronic fatigue, mental-emotional disturbances, hearing, or disease.

The school nurse uses the professional reports from doctors and dentists on corrections or treatment of students as a firm evaluative device. Health appraisals require interpretation of the results of measurement. School nurses keep the administrator and other school personnel informed regarding health problems. Furthermore, the school nurse interprets the school health program, facilities, and policies to families and the community; success is often measured by how effectively the school nurse relates to parents.

Another common device for measuring health outcome is the survey. This may involve the community or the school alone for health information. Surveys can reveal the need for health teaching, and pupils may be involved for the tally, observations, and interviews.

Health education

There is so much new knowledge and it constantly changes. The school nurse may assist in planning the curriculum for health instruction, and, of course, the nurse has used health services as a means of direct and indirect teaching, but as

---

[3]Lampe, J. M.: Early identification of the "at risk" child, J. Sch. Health 42:214, 1972.

described by Bernard H. McKenna,[4] it is next to impossible to relate learning outcomes to teaching performance. He further states:

> Evaluation is a complicated activity, difficult to conceptualize fully in all its ramifications and even more difficult to implement with sound substance and fair process. Help to become involved in:
> building understanding about evaluation
> selecting evaluation instruments
> training in the use of evaluation instruments
> planning in-service education based on results of evaluation

Tests and evaluation of health knowledge are more meaningful when they relate directly to the class; however, there are standardized health knowledge tests available for elementary school use, as summarized by Carl Willgoose.[5] He likewise has given examples of tests used for health attitudes and habits that are more difficult to construct. However, a more effective method of teaching is the self-testing evaluation. A pupil may rate himself on a checklist of health expectancies and these decisions can show growth of attitudes toward the items checked.

Studies for appraising health-related attitudes show that positive attitudes are necessary for the application of knowledge toward improving health behavior. The latest large-scale study of student needs and interests was published in 1969.[6] This research indicates that students' needs are unmet. Educators at all levels are failing to provide for student health education needs and are therefore turning students into society who are not able or prepared to resolve the health problems generated by our contemporary life-style. We need to consider what the student wants to know.

The school nurse participates in public relations and interprets the school health program to school and community groups. An aid in the evaluative questionnaire is the parent interview. Habits and attitudes pertinent to home and the school health instruction can show evaluative improvement. Parents often say, "You teach him how to brush his teeth and he does it, but we are ignored at home."

We have mentioned evaluative tests of (1) health knowledge, (2) health attitudes and habits, and (3) self-test activities. The results of these tests are more revealing when combined with teachers' observations.

PLANNING OUTCOMES

School health services and school nursing programs, in almost every instance and in almost every community, outrun and outlive staff and facilities and surely remain in practice long after they have been proved unnecessary. Since much school nursing practice is outdated, either in developing a new service or redirecting an established one, it is usually wise to establish priorities when setting up a service and incorporate some means of evaluating and redirecting services at regular intervals.

---

[4]McKenna, Bernard H.: Teacher evaluation—some implications, Today's Education, p. 55, 1973.

[5]Willgoose, Carl E.: Health education in the elementary school, Philadelphia, 1966, W. B. Saunders Co.

[6]Byler, Ruth, Lewis, Gertrude, and Totman, Ruth: Teach us what we want to know, Mental Health Materials Center, 1969, The Connecticut State Board of Education.

What about routine checking of height and weight? Dental inspection? Routine physical examinations? Health education as rainy day health instruction? Testing vision and hearing every year? A look at current literature and recent research not only in school health but in public health, medicine, education, and the behavioral sciences gives excellent clues to new approaches to these practices, methods for setting priorities, and means of evaluation. A little experimentation and careful evaluation of results will probably mean improved health services for more children. Neglect of selected outdated practices pays dividends in released nurse time for more meaningful activities.

Selective neglect

The "theory of selective neglect" is a term borrowed from a good friend, B. Otis Cobb, M.D., Professor in Pediatrics at the University of California at Davis. He is one of the strongest supporters of school health and one of its greatest critics.

The theory of selective neglect is the simple process of deciding what is most important to do on the job for each day, or each week, or each month, or each year, or in future program planning. This means that a plan or program is made with conscious or unconscious objectives, priorities, and hopefuly some means of evaluating this plan. This also means that certain activities are not done and that persons involved in the work are well aware of this. For example, a school nurse has a plan to test eyes or do a classroom demonstration on the hazards of smoking for a certain day at her school. She is going to "neglect" her immunization program, her routine drop-in trade, records, and a group conference on a child in a special class because she knows she cannot do everything and spread herself so that nothing gets done well.

At the policy and program level this same concept holds true. No program is ever ideal in this age of shortages of finances and trained personnel. Hopefully at this level a review of records and reports will give clues to where many activities are just busywork for the nurses, probably instigated years ago by someone with a pet theory or interest. These are oversimplified examples of selective neglect.

Setting priorities

If every school nursse in the country would take time to list her total activities and then have a variety of persons rate these actiivties according to the health needs of their school and community, it would facilitate defining workable objectives (not so vague that they are meaningless) in setting priorities and "neglecting" certain age-old practices. It might be something like the boxed material on p. 141.

In considering the evaluation for vision screening, the nurse might find that while many defects are being discovered, the number of referrals is very small and an even smaller number is being evaluated by an eye specialist. It also might become evident that the nurse is identifying many more children with known defects who have been referred for care but are counted each year as having identified vision defects. Wouldn't it be an improved practice to screen less often and offer better follow-up and/or give the nurse more time for other programs?

If it is the practice of the school ophthalmologist to review the records of all pupils failing the Snellen test before referring a child to an eye specialist, perhaps

Activity	Why and whom	Where and when	Priority*	How to evaluate
Vision screening	State law—local practice	Retest every 3 years	1	Study law—research in frequency and types of vision problems
		Test new pupils yearly	10	
	Scheduling and preparation of class	Nurse's office	3	
	Done by volunteers	Classroom	1	Number of defects New Known
	Rechecked by nurse	Nurse's office	2	Number of referrals
	Records reviewed by school ophthalmologist before referral for care	Nurse's office	10	Number of referrals completed

*Range of 1-10; 1 is highest priority, 10 is lowest priority.

there is too much time being spent on this process. Is it really necessary for the ophthalmologist to review cases? Isn't this a waste of trained professional personnel performing tasks that could be "neglected" or done by less qualified workers? Wouldn't vision screening be a more meaningful program if vision testing were done every three years, plus referrals by teachers and all new students, so the school nurse could have more time to work with pupils, parents, and local sources of care to get the discovered defects corrected?

If volunteers are used in the screening program, are they well supervised? Could they have more responsibility? As in all other areas of school nursing, setting priorities, except at the health office level, must be a group process.

Nurses must evaluate their programs. This will mean change and perhaps compromise on established practices, which is not easy. This type of activity has been too long in coming to school health programs. It has been part of business and industry procedure for years and more recently is being adapted in some public health programs.

TIME AND ACTIVITY STUDIES*

Another tool in evaluating programs, nurse performance, and setting priorities is the use of a time and activity study. Usually these are short-term processes and

*Excerpted with minor modifications from Bryan, Doris S., and Cook, Thelma S.: Redirection of school nursing services in culturally deprived neighborhoods, Oakland Unified School District, Final Report, 1968.

give many clues as to what activities the staff is spending time on, where cuts would be profitable, and what areas of the program should be increased. The following is one used in the *Redirection Study* cited many times before:

Instructions for use of the Daily Time and Activity Study Report form

The Daily Time and Activity Study Report form will be carried out during the following statistical months:

Second statistical month	20 school days
Fifth statistical month	20 school days
Seventh statistical month	20 school days
Ninth statistical month	20 school days
Second statistical month	20 school days
Fifth statistical month	20 school days
Seventh statistical month	15 school days
Ninth statistical month	20 school days

Each school nurse and paraprofessional will complete, independently, a Daily Time and Activity Study Report form *for each workday* in the time study periods. The completed forms may be turned in on a daily basis, if this is more convenient, but they *must* be turned in on a weekly basis. All forms *must* be in on the last day of each of the time study periods.

Forms must be complete. Forms must be accurate!

Counting time. All time for a given workday is to be indicated *in minutes* in the space provided for each activity category. Each person completing the report will be responsible for giving *total time* for a given day *in minutes*.

Total time for a school nurse should equal at least 435 ± 15 minutes for each workday. If a school nurse attends evening meetings, etc., or works more than a 7¼-hour day, this should be included for the daily report, and the total time therefore would be increased accordingly. Coffee time and lunch time should be shown in space provided unless school business was conducted while having coffee or lunch and, in this case, time would be indicated for the appropriate activity.

Total time for a paraprofessional should equal 450 ± 15 minutes. Coffee breaks and lunch time need not be indicated, since it is not anticipated that the paraprofessional will conduct school business at these times.

DIRECT SERVICES TO STUDENTS

Under Direct Services to Students, the number of times a given service was provided during the day is needed and this should be given in the column provided. Include travel time as part of the time spent providing the service or attending the function for which it was incurred. Most items are self-explanatory, but the following *added* explanations should be carefully noted.

Care for accidents and emergency illness

Include under Nursing Care and Follow-up Activities *all* time spent in providing needed care, communicating with the teacher, principal, parent, or other interested parties, and any other related activities.

If the child is transported home, include travel time and conferencing with parent in the category Transporting Child Home.

All time spent in unsuccessful attempts to reach parents should be accounted for under Unsuccessful Attempts to Reach Parents.

DAILY TIME AND ACTIVITY STUDY REPORT FORM

Name _____ School _____ Date _____

TIME IN
MINUTES   NO.   SERVICES AND ACTIVITIES

DIRECT SERVICES TO STUDENTS

Care for accidents and emergency illness

Nursing care and follow-up activities

Transporting child home

Unsuccessful attempts to reach parents

Maintenance of emergency file

Other:

Care for children with other immediate problems

Nursing care and follow-up activities

Transporting child home

Unsuccessful attempts to reach parents

Other:

Children paying a social call

**Service to children having an attendance problem
and the nonreturns**

Home visit

Other contacts with parents

Unsuccessful attempts to reach parents

Contact with school personnel

Other:

Health appraisal activities

Health appraisal reports

Observation of pupil health (group situations)

Planned teacher-nurse conference

Initial classroom vision screening

Vision retest

Audiometric screening

Examination by school physician

Weighing and measuring

Special services referral

Other:

STUDENT SAMPLE		OTHER THAN STUDENT SAMPLE		
TIME IN MINUTES	NO.	TIME IN MINUTES	NO.	SERVICES AND ACTIVITIES
				Individual child health supervision
				Conference or communication with—
				Teacher or principal
				Other school personnel
				Community agency
				Source of medical care
				Contact with students
				Contact with parents
				Home
				School
				Written
				Phone
				Making appointment for nursing conference
				Case conference
				Making appointment for student
				Unsuccessful attempts to reach parents
				Immunizations
				Service to a family member
				Transporting and accompanying child to source of medical care
				School lunch program
				Other:
				Student records and special reports
				Review and/or updating records on transfers
				Tracing students and/or student records
				Maintenance of health records
				Maintenance of defect cards
				Preparation of special referrals and reports
				Record review and planning follow-up
				Other:

TIME IN
MINUTES   SERVICES AND ACTIVITIES

ORGANIZATION, PLANNING, AND ADMINISTRATION OF SCHOOL HEALTH PROGRAM

Overall planning and administration activities

With principal

With other school personnel

Nurse helpers

Independently

Attendance at faculty meetings

Participation in PTA or parent group activities

Maintenance of nurse's office

Maintenance of first-aid supplies in classroom

Maintaining good interpersonal relations

Reading school mail and communications

Faculty social functions

Special school activities and functions

Other:

NURSING ADMINISTRATION AND PROFESSIONAL GROWTH

Nursing staff meetings

Attending the professional meetings

Nursing committee assignments

Administrative reports

Conferences with supervisor

Contacts with nursing office

Participation in student nurse program

Orientation of new employees

Orientation of visitors

Other:

PARTICIPATION IN COMMUNITY ACTIVITIES
Explain:

TIME IN
MINUTES   SERVICES AND ACTIVITIES

MAINTENANCE OF HEALTHFUL SCHOOL ENVIRONMENT

Activities related to safe and healthful physical environment

Individual health counseling provided to teacher or school personnel

Direct care provided to sick or injured member of school staff

Communicable disease control

Other:

HEALTH EDUCATION

Prescreening health educational activities

Participation in classroom instruction

Bulletin boards, displays, and exhibits

Consultation to teachers

Special projects or activities

Special educational programs on health for parents

Health educational materials

Other (explain):

ABSENT FROM DUTY

OTHER ACTIVITIES

Lunch

Coffee

Assisting in school office

Other (explain):

Total minutes for day
Time began workday _____
Time ended workday _____

Care for children with other immediate problems

Include in this category the time spent providing care to individual children who are not sick but who are sent to the nurse because they have problems of a self-limited nature that require time and attention of someone in their management.

Include under Nursing Care and Follow-up Activities *all* time spent in providing needed care, communicating with teacher, principal, parent, or other interested parties, and any other related activities.

If the child is transported home, include travel time and conferring with parent in the category Transporting Child Home.

All time spent in unsuccessful attempts to reach parents should be accounted for under Unsuccessful Attempts to Reach Parents.

Health appraisal activities

Health appraisal reports

Include all time spent on health inventory, medical examination, and dental examination reports, except recording on Health Record. This includes distribution, collection, review, sending letters or notes home concerning these forms, etc.

Transcribing findings from these reports on the Health Record should be accounted for under Maintenance of Health Record.

Initial classroom vision screening

Include time spent in preparation for as well as actual screening time.
Include both Snellen and color vision test.
Include vision testing of youngsters new to the school and special referrals.

Vision retest

Include time spent in preparation for as well as actual screening time.

Audiometric screening program activities

Include all time spent in relation to initial screening and retest of students.

Examination by school physician

Include all time spent in preparing for visit by school physician—selection of students, notification of teacher, parent, and pupil records—as well as actual conference time.

Weighing and measuring

If weighing and measuring are done as a health appraisal activity for the Other than Student Sample, include all time spent in planning and carrying out the procedure under Health Appraisal Activities.

If weighing and measuring are done as part of a health educational project, include under Health Education, Special Projects or Activities.

If weighing and measuring are done as a part of a special health appraisal activity for the student sample, include under Child Health Supervision, Student Sample, Contact with Student.

Special services referral

Include all time spent in Health Appraisal Activities in preparation of referring an individual student to the school district division of special services.

Other

Explain, giving time.

Individual child supervision

Include here those services provided to or in behalf of students for health promotional reasons or because a child has a special health problem and/or defect that requires nursing supervision. Examples of defects: vision defects, hearing losses, or other physical defects; poor health habits that require counseling and guidance from nurse; dietary problems. All individual student follow-up activities beyond the initial screening activities should be included here.

It is understood that the service which a school nurse provides on home visits or conferences with parents at school is family centered. Therefore, for example, in a conference with a parent, any or all of the following might take place: A definite service or general health teaching may be provided in behalf of a member of the "student sample" group; a definite service may be provided to siblings who fall into the "other than student sample group"; a definite service may be provided to another member of the family; and some general health teaching may occur that is directed at the entire family as a group, such as beginning each day with a well-balanced breakfast for all family members, having a plan for medical care in case of emergency or sudden illness for all members of the family, or up-to-date immunizations for all family members. To eliminate confusion in the completion of the time study form, some general rules need to be followed:

1. Time spent providing a specific service to a member of the "student sample" group for a specific problem or the general health teaching and counseling service that has been set up in the project for this group should be accounted for in the student sample category. It is expected that the nursing service will be family centered and all members of the family will hopefully receive some benefit from the service. As long as there has been no specific family member specific problem-centered service, charge up all time to "student sample" under Child Health Supervision and a count of "1" in the "No." column.
2. The same reasoning, as outlined in number one above, would hold true when visiting a member of the "other than student sample" group.
3. If a nurse makes a home visit or has a conference with a parent for the purpose of providing service to members of both the "student sample" and "other than student sample" groups, time and number of services will need to be appropriately accounted for in both of these categories.
4. Time spent providing service specifically to a family member (or household member) for a specific problem, should be accounted for in Service to a Family Member under Child Health Supervision with the number of persons to be served in the "No." column.

If a nurse-parent conference was held at the time of registration of the student (not student registration per se), this should be counted under Contact with Parents—School.

Immunizations

Include all time spent in assessing immunization needs, making referrals, etc., including polio and polio exclusion letters.

Student records and special reports

Preparation of special referrals and reports

Include all time spent in the preparation of necessary reports to facilitate needed care— medical examination, medical care, or service from the schools, special services. Include Obtaining Medical resumes, Ear Center report, Request for Special Service, Application for Home Instruction, Application for Special Class, etc.

Maintenance of health records

Include *all* time spent in the maintenance of this record.

Maintenance of defect cards

Include *all* time spent in initiating and maintaining this record.

ORGANIZATION, PLANNING, AND ADMINISTRATION OF THE SCHOOL HEALTH PROGRAM
Attendance at PTA or parent meetings

If conducting or carrying out an educational program, count time under Health Education, PTA Programs on Health.

Maintenance of nurse's office

Include time spent ordering and maintaining supplies, maintaining first-aid tray, answering phone, and taking messages by nurse assistant, etc.

Special school activities and functions

Include time spent in such activities as watching or participating in Halloween parade, school play, Christmas program, school committee assignments unrelated to health or health education, etc.

NURSING ADMINISTRATION AND PROFESSIONAL GROWTH
Nursing staff meetings

Include time spent in attending regular staff meetings as well as special meetings that may be called from time to time.

Administrative reports

If reports are brought into the health services office, include travel and delivery time here also as well as time spent in preparation of reports.

Contact with health services office

Include time spent contacting nursing office, as well as time spent for the sole purpose of coming in for paycheck.

MAINTENANCE OF A HEALTHFUL SCHOOL ENVIRONMENT
Activities related to safe and healthful physical environment

Include participation in the detection and/or elimination of any hazardous condition—safety hazards, improper lighting, heating, or ventilation problems, sanitation problems, etc. Include fire drill and civil defense drills here.

Communicable disease control

Include all items related to communicable disease control, except for immunizations, which have been included under Individual Child Health Supervision.

Other

Explain, giving time.

HEALTH EDUCATION
Prescreening health educational activities

Include time spent in preparation.

Consultation to teachers

Include consultation regarding health education materials, teaching units on health displays, or projects related to health, etc.

Special projects or activities

Give one sentence explaining activity.

PTA programs on health

Include preparation time.

Health education materials

Include all time spent ordering, maintaining, and distributing health education materials, including films.

OTHER ACTIVITIES

Assisting in school office

Include time spent here assisting school secretary or assisting with school office activities.

Include time spent assisting with student registration activities. Health conferences conducted at the time of registration, however, should be acounted for under Child Health Supervision, Contact with Parent at School.

Other

Include all time spent in other activities not accounted for elsewhere and explain.

EVALUATION OF PERSONNEL*

Regardless of program planning and evaluation, setting priorities and implementation of programs depend on the competence and dedication of the personnel. Identical programs may be outstanding successes or complete failures, depending on the persons involved.

There are many performance appraisals, but often in the school setting these evaluations are designed for teachers and only adapted for school health personnel. The health worker must know early in the school year how he will be evaluated—hopefully based on the objectives, goals, and job expectations. In more recent evaluations, they are set up jointly between the administrator or nursing supervisor and include measurement techniques for performance expectations.

Appraisal for individual school nurse performance

The Individual School Nurse Performance Appraisal was developed for use in the project *Redirection of School Nursing Services in Culturally Deprived Neighborhoods* as a mechanism to aid both program development and individual school nurse development in the experimental schools.

AGENCY GOALS, THE SCHOOL NURSE, THE SCHOOL
NURSE SUPERVISOR, AND EVALUATION

An esssential ingredient of every organization is a goal or set of goals toward which it is to advance and by which, ultimately, it evaluates itself as well as is evaluated by others whom it serves. The performance appraisal of employees in the pursuit of the identified goals is an integral part of this evaluation process.[7]

---

*Excerpted with minor modifications from Bryan, Doris S., and Cook, Thelma S.: Redirection of school nursing services in culturally deprived neighborhoods, Oakland Unified School District, Final Report, 1968.

[7]Shanks, Mary D., and Kennedy, Dorothy A.: The theory and practice of nursing service administration, New York, 1965, McGraw-Hill Book Co., Inc.

The importance of the individual employee to the achievement of specified agency goals no doubt varies from discipline to discipline, from agency to agency, and among the various disciplines within different agencies. Hanlon[8] points out that in the field of public health (which holds equally true for the school nurse) to an unusually high degree the personnel are, as a whole, the health department. Their behavior and successful functioning determine, in the final analysis, the acceptance and success of the organization's work. It is through the personal contacts of the staff that health program activities are carried out and success depends upon the acceptance and reaction of those who are served.

Nursing administrators and supervisors have as an ultimate goal the fusing of two major forces:

1. The potential that a nurse brings with her to the job
2. The goals that the organization has set and the creative use of nursing skills in the achievement of these goals

The nurse brings with her to her job her own personal goals, individual reasons for seeking employment, aptitude, a highly personalized source of motivation, an equally individualized criteria by which the nurse measures success, and the nurse's own individual concept of and expectations of nursing.

The nurse administrator or supervisor is ever seeking the right formula that will yield the optimum in the employee-agency relationship—that is, achieving the goals of the employing organization while at the same time assisting in the creation of a climate in which the individual nurse will find a fulfillment of the nurse's individual needs. The performance evaluation or rating can be a tool to determine if the desired dynamic equilibrium has been achieved in the employer-employee relationship.[9, 10]

The school nurse administrator or supervisor carries the responsibility to appraise the performance of staff. A climate in which a *cooperative* evaluation takes place between supervisor and staff is desirable. Evaluation of individual performance should be done in accordance with established criteria.[11]

CHECKLIST FOR SCHOOL NURSE PERFORMANCE

The School Nurse Performance Appraisal Checklist was developed to be used by the school nurse supervisor in conjunction with the established evaluation instrument adopted for use by the Oakland Public Schools, *Guide for the Evaluation and Improvement of Professional Services*.[12] The latter contains a scale along with criteria to be followed for the rating of all professionals employed by the school district —teachers, school nurses, etc. The school district is interested in selecting and re-

[8]Hanlon, John J.: Principles of public health administration, St. Louis, 1960, The C. V. Mosby Co.

[9]Blum, Henrik L., and Leonard, Alvin R.: Public administration—a public health viewpoint, New York, 1963, The Macmillan Co.

[10]Pfiffner, John M., and Sherwood, Frank P.: Administrative organization, Englewood Cliffs, N. J., 1960, Prentice-Hall, Inc.

[11]Freeman, Ruth, and Holmes, Edward: Administration of public health service, Philadelphia, 1960, W. B. Saunders Co.

[12]Oakland Public Schools: Guide for the evaluation and improvement of professional services, Administrative bulletin 12, Oakland Public Schools, 1966.

taining the best teachers possible for its young people, and the form and procedure used is designed toward this end. The School Nurse Performance Appraisal Checklist allows for a very active participation by each staff school nurse in the nurse's own individual appraisal as well as an ongoing assessment and was designed primarily with the following objectives in mind:

1. To provide the nurse with the incentive, as well as the opportunity, to exercise initiative and creative ability in developing and implementing a school health program in the nurse's individual school
2. To emphasize the responsibility that each nurse carries for the development and implementation of the health program in the nurse's school and each nurse's own individual performance
3. To provide the supervisor with an opportunity of assessing the various levels of performance by the staff and to identify with the staff areas where staff education and in-service programs are needed
4. To assist in the development of the nursing program for each individual school as well as for the total school district
5. To hopefully develop a climate that will encourage critical thinking by each school nurse about the nurse's school nursing program and invite each nurse to actively participate in planning for changes that may be indicated

NECESSARY CONDITIONS

1. The department of health services has established goals toward which the nurse is expected to work and to achieve and that these goals have been communicated to the school nurse.[13]
2. School nurses understand their job and the relative importance of its components.[13]
3. The school nurses come to the district well qualified. However, it is recognized that individual performance will vary from nurse to nurse and will be greatly dependent upon individual areas of skill, levels of knowledge, personal interests, prior experience, etc.
4. School nurses, granted, have personal reasons and personal goals that are basic to their reasons for employment; however, they assume responsibility for the quality and quantity of their performance and are actively interested, as professionals, and as indicated by their behavior, in the development of the nursing service through self-development and change, as indicated and made necessary by the changing needs of the school community they serve as well as new knowledge available.

METHOD

Step I. At the beginning of the school year, nurses should review their total school health programs, clarifying with their principals and the supervisor of nursing services any questions relative to the job for which they are to be held accountable.

Step II. Individual school nurses identify within their school health programs

---

[13]Oakland Public Schools: Role and function of the nurse in the Oakland Public Schools, Administrative bulletin 23, Oakland Public Schools, 1964.

at least one, or more depending on the nurse, personal goals (targets or end points) toward which they would like to work or emphasize during the immediate school year. The goal could well be one involving one or more of the broad, major functional areas of nursing:

1. Assessing
2. Planning
3. Implementing
4. Evaluating
5. Study and research[14]

The goal, or goals, should be well identified, realistic in the school setting, and both manageable and challenging from the point of view of the nurse. Some examples of such goals might be as follows:

1. To make a careful review or take a critical look at the current method or methods used by the school nurse to make an individual assessment of the health status of entering students—the "what" that is being done, and the reasons why it is done, the effectiveness of the method, and recommendations that the nurse might have for change
2. To explore both the need for and interest in developing a parent education program in healthful living practices for parents of kindergarten children and to begin to develop such a program if indicated

The goal, on the other hand, might well be a special project that the nurse has designed and wishes to carry out.

Step III. The personal goal or goals are discussed with the principal and supervisor of nursing services. This could well be done along with step I above.

Step IV. Evaluation using the School Nurse Performance Appraisal Checklist could be held at the termination of the school year by nurse, principal, and school nurse supervisor, or evaluation could be at specified intervals during the year, depending on the need and desire of those concerned.

Step V. The following could be natural outcomes of the evaluation conferences:

1. Revision of nursing program where necessary and re-setting of nursing goals
2. Identification by the school nurse supervisor of areas where in-service education might be desired by staff

Evaluation method of the performance of the paraprofessional[15]

The paraprofessional has been assigned and trained to perform, under the supervision of the school nurse and direction of the school administrator, selected technical skills that heretofore have been performed by the school nurse. This has been done for the expressed purpose of releasing school nurses in order that they might be redirected into more fruitful areas of service that require their specialized knowledge and skills.

---

[14]American Nurses' Association: Functions and qualifications for school nurses, New York, 1966, The Association.

[15]This method of evaluating the performance of the paraprofessional is an adaptation of "A Method for Rating the Proficiency of the Hospital General Staff Nurse, Manual of Directions," published by Research and Studies Service, National League for Nursing, 1964, Code no. 19-1122.

It is essential to have an adequate method of assessing performance in order to be assured that the duties performed are done so with the degree of knowledge and skill required by the school district. This evaluation is much more detailed than the School Nurse Performance Appraisal.

PERFORMANCE AREAS

The paraprofessionals are evaluated on a nine-point scale in each of eight performance areas. Except for performance area VIII, the evaluation will be directed toward their performance of specific duties assigned in each area, which they carry out under the direction and supervision of the school nurse. These performance areas are as follows:

    I. Maintenance of school nurse's office
   II. Individual child care
 III. Health appraisal activities
 IV. Individual child health supervision
   V. Records and reports
 VI. Health education
VII. Other clerical duties as may be assigned
VIII. Job approach

SPECIFIC DUTIES ASSIGNED IN EACH PERFORMANCE AREA

Performance area I—maintenance of nurse's office

1. Keeps the health office attractive and in order at all times.
2. Participates in the ordering and maintenance of supplies.
3. Answers phone and takes messages for nurse in nurse's absence.
4. Keeps first-aid tray ready for use at all times.
5. Maintains emergency file.
6. Maintains first-aid supplies in individual classrooms.

Performance area II—individual child care

Greets all students who come to the nurse's office seeking assistance, assesses their individual needs, and provides care as needed or refers to the school nurse or principal as needed.

1. Renders *minor* first aid and care of *minor* emergency illness in accordance with established policy.
2. Refers to the school nurse those pupils who need more extensive nursing care and follow-up.
3. Seeks guidance from school nurse when in doubt as to what action she should take.
4. Under the direction of the school principal, follows the Exclusion from School procedure as outlined in the School Nursing Procedure Manual.
5. Transports sick or injured pupils home as may be necessary.

Performance area III—participation in health appraisal activities

1. Vision screening
   a. Performs initial vision screening tests on children in designated grades,

children new to the district, and special referrals by parent or school personnel.

   b. Refers to the school nurse all pupils who fail the initial screening test.

   c. May do vision retest on students as directed by school nurse.

   d. For the less severe visual defects, may participate in selected follow-up activities as directed by the school nurse such as:

      (1.) Completion of Referral for Eye Examination

      (2.) Phone conference with parent

      (3.) Note or conference with teacher regarding results of vision test and eye examiner's recommendations.

   e. Records vision screening results, follow-up activities, and eye examinations on appropriate reports.

2. School physician examination and conference or comprehensive screening program

   a. Participates in the scheduling activities of youngsters. Notifies teachers and parents of appointment time.

   b. Assists as needed on the day of examination.

   c. Sees that student's Cumulative Health Record is in order prior to the examination and that all necessary record work is completed following the examination.

3. Audiometric screening program

   a. Participates in carrying out nursing responsibilities as outlined in the school nursing manual under Hearing Program, as directed by school nurse. Records threshold test results and summary of medical findings on Cumulative Health Record.

4. Health inventories, health examination, and dental examination reports

   a. Assists in the distribution and collection of health appraisal forms.

   b. May assist parent at the time of registration in the completion of the Health Inventory form and discusses with the parent the importance of the completion of the medical and dental examinations.

   c. Reviews health inventories upon their return, referring to the school nurse all pupils needing special follow-up as indicated by the reports.

   d. Records on appropriate records and files in pupil's cumulative folder.

Performance area IV—individual child health supervision

1. Communicable disease—prevention

   a. Polio—follows the procedure for implementing polio programs as outlined in nursing manual.

   b. Other preventable diseases—appraises immunization needs of pupils (by review of Health Record) and initiates Disease Protection Reminder. Telephone calls may be made to the parent either to assess immunization needs or to make referrals as indicated.

2. Makes appointments for students as directed by the school nurse.

3. Does follow-up on selected absentees and nonreturns as may be delegated by the school nurse. Home visits may be made by the nurse assistant if so directed.

Performance area V—student records and special reports

1. Assists in the maintenance of the individual Cumulative Health Record, recording pertinent data from health appraisal forms, vision screening results, etc.
2. Assists in the initiation of and maintenance of defect cards.
3. Reviews cumulative folders on transfer, updating records on students who are leaving the school and referring to the nurse incoming students who have health problems.
4. Assists in the preparation of special referrals and reports as delegated by school nurse.
5. Completes departmental and evaluation reports as delegated by nurse.
6. Traces students and student records as necessary.

Performance area VI—health education

1. Orders, maintains, and distributes health education material as directed by nurse.
2. Maintains bulletin board in nurse's office.
3. Assists nurse in special educational projects conducted by school nurse.

Performance area VII—other clerical duties as may be assigned

1. Assists in registration of students.
2. Prepares special notices as may be directed by the school nurse.
3. Maintenance of health records and preparation of reports for which adequate provision has not been made in other specific performance areas.

Performance area VIII—job approach

To be considered in the overall job approach: interpersonal relations, initiative, dependability, conduct, personal appearance, attendance, punctuality, cooperation, interest in job, and attitude.

RATING SCALE

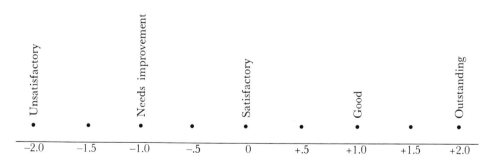

Unsatisfactory

1. Requires constant guidance and instruction.
2. Cannot be depended on to carry out assignments unsupervised.

3. Cannot be depended on to provide individual child care or carry out approved first-aid and emergency practices with safety or required skill.
4. Cannot be depended on to carry out other selected technical duties completely or adequately, without frequent mishap or error.
5. Does not understand the scope and function of the position.
6. Has difficulty in "carry-over" from orientation and in-service educational meetings to "on-the-job" performance.

Needs improvement

1. Needs frequent, direct guidance and detailed instructions to prevent mishap or error in carrying out selected technical duties.
2. Is able to provide direct care to students and can carry out approved first-aid and emergency practices with necessary skill and safety, *but requires intensive supervision.*
3. May be unsure of the total scope and function of the position and has difficulty in interpreting the position accurately.

Satisfactory

1. Carries out selected technical duties assigned with safety, sufficient skill, and with minimal error or mishap, but requires a reasonable amount of supervision and direction.
2. Understands and is able to carry out accident and emergency policy with reasonable skill and safety.
3. Understands the scope and function of the position.
4. Is able to assess, with reasonable accuracy, the needs of the individual students who are referred to the nurse and act accordingly.
5. Is dependable.

Good

1. Is able to carry out selected technical duties assigned with safety, with better than average skill, and with minimal error or mishap.
2. Understands and is able to carry out policy for accident and emergency illness with the safety and skill required.
3. Is able to function with a minimal amount of guidance.
4. Is able to carry over from one learning situation to another.
5. Assumes responsibility and is capable of some independent planning.
6. Understands the scope and function of the position and is able to interpret the position to school personnel and parents when indicated.

Outstanding

1. Consistently maintains a high level of performance.
2. Has unusual self-direction.
3. Assumes responsibility within the scope and function of the position and does some independent planning.
4. Needs minimal supervision but does require guidance and instruction in the complex or unique situations.

5. Exercises good judgment in assessing the needs of the individual students and provision of direct child care.
6. Understands the scope and function of the position and can be depended on to interpret this accurately to school personnel, parents, and other interested persons should the occasion arise.
7. Is of help to project staff in the development and further refinement of the position.

SUMMARY REPORT

A single-page summary report, showing an average rating for each of the eight performance areas and containing a summary statement by the school nurse, nurse assistant, and project coordinator will be completed at the end of the evaluation period.

Objectives to be achieved

1. To obtain a descriptive report, or a cumulative picture, of the performance of the nurse assistant from which and through which an evaluation of their performance might be made
2. To provide a method by which the actual observations of their behavior might be classified, to provide a stimulus for observing all areas of performance, and to provide a means of evaluation based on facts and observations rather than on generalizations and opinions
3. Hopefully, to provide a means of collecting data from which an inference might be made with respect to the adequacy of quality of performance of the nurse assistant; hopefully also, to gather data that will assist in the determination of the true contribution which the nurse assistant makes to the total school health program

The procedure

1. Each school-community nurse will be provided with an Evaluation of Performance that contains a rating scale for each of the eight performance areas to be evaluated and a summary report. There will be adequate orientation of the staff involved.
2. The evaluation period will be one semester in length. During this period of time, the school-community nurses may plan for specific time periods when they will observe the paraprofessionals performing their assigned duties, or this may be an ongoing type operation. Observations should be made on different days of the week, at different hours of the day, when the workload is both heavy and light, and covering all performance areas. Multiple observations should be made in each area to be evaluated.
3. School-community nurses should record their observations in the form of *brief* descriptive sentences, yet provide clear understanding to them when they refer back to the report at a later date. Observations should be numbered —1, 2, 3, etc.—in the order that they are made and the date of observation included. There should be several descriptions for each performance area to be rated.

EVALUATION OF PARAPROFESSIONAL

PERFORMANCE AREA I*

Maintenance of nurse's office

Rating scale

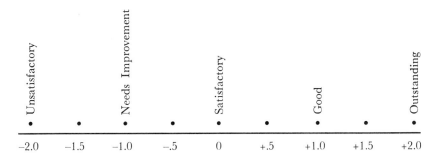

Observations:

Observations should be numbered in the order that they are made and the date of the observation included. (Use other side of page, if necessary.)

Are the above observations typical of the usual behavior?

What have been the special counseling needs?

*Evaluation form can be used for each of the eight performance areas by changing the title.

4. Once an observation is written down, it is ready for rating by writing the number of the observation on the scale line of the given performance area.
5. At the end of the observational period, a visual average is made of the ratings in each given performance area and transferred to the summary sheet.
6. A final evaluation of the performance of the nurse assistant is then made with the necessary conferencing.

Problems inherent in the method

1. The method is subjective, although effort has been made to be somewhat objective, analytical, and thorough.
2. Other than for the limited definitions assigned to the scale, there are no statements of criteria or norms to guide the evaluators in their assessment of the paraprofessional.
3. The individual value systems of the school nurses, project coordinator, and project director will greatly influence not only *what* is observed but also the *interpretation* of the observed.
4. The paraprofessionals, in working in close association with and under the direct supervision of their respective school nurse, have to some degree patterned their behavior after the nurse to whom assigned and assumed some of the nurse's values in the area of the work to be done and the performance of that work. This, no doubt, will influence how the school nurse rates the paraprofessional's performance. In turn, nursing supervisors must make provision for the individual impact of the school nurse upon the paraprofessional when making their evaluation.

Justification for use of method. The position of the paraprofessional is a new and developing one. There are no stated criteria or stated norms of performance which can be applied at the present time.

EVALUATION—AN ONGOING PROCESS

There needs to be a look to the future, an awareness of the trend for health instruction, which is so well told by Jerrold S. Greenberg.[16] He lists eight emerging concepts:

1. Accountability
2. Behavioral objectives
3. Performance contracting
4. Voucher system
5. Differentiated staffing
6. School without walls
7. Sensitivity training
8. Methodologies

He also believes that all of these concepts in schooling have implications for health instruction. Furthermore, he says, "Health educators' concerns for attitudinal de-

---

[16]Greenberg, Jerrold S.: Emerging educational concepts and health instruction, J. Sch. Health **42**:356, 1972.

velopment would seem to indicate a need for increased variety in learning experiences."

Another study tells us that no screening procedure or combination of procedures can detect each and every variation from the normal that may exist; screening procedures detect only those health defects they are designed to find. Therefore every health assessment program needs an open-ended procedure that will pick up unexpected defects.[17]

How evaluative techniques are used is more important than the tests themselves. There are reasons for meeting the expectations of an evaluation:

1. It may provide opportunity to assist teachers with scientifically accurate health material.
2. It affords opportunity to observe the school environment and report health and safety hazards to the school administrator.
3. It presents an opportunity to interpret the scope and significance of immunizations to school personnel, parents, and pupils.
4. It provides nurses the chance to counsel with parents regarding health of their children, helps the family accept the responsibility for providing care, and helps them make use of available health facilities.
5. It assists students by stimulating behavior modification and helps them to accept and adjust positively to their physical limitations.
6. It can keep communication lines open and acquaint the school personnel with resources of the community and vice versa and creates in the community an awareness of the health needs of schoolchildren. It also fosters communication with community agencies, with physicians, and with dentists.
7. It uses health services as a means of direct and indirect teaching. The school nurse assumes the responsibility for interpreting health needs of pupils for health instruction.
8. It identifies health problems through health appraisal and screening programs.
9. It demonstrates the school nurse's competencies in all situations. It represents the nurse using critical judgment and discrete observation to evaluate symptoms and referral needs.
10. It furthers the health program by stimulating utilization of current research and continuing in-service education.

SUMMARY MODEL

It is important to develop a plan to evaluate the objectives and standards of performance for student progress and professional competence. Evaluation plan I can be used to examine school personnel in areas such as the provision of school nurse services, school health screening, referrals, follow-up, health education, policy recommendations, and process control (Figs. 8-1 to 8-7). Performance criteria represent the degree to which a particular school population is expected to attain the

---

[17]Eisner, Victor, and Oglesby, Allan: Health assessment of children. VIII. The unexpected health defect, J. Sch. Health **42:**348, 1972.

Text continued on p. 169.

Evaluation Plan I

Objectives and Standards of Performance
for Student Progress and Professional Competence

Toda, Mary F.	Durant School	1972-73
Certificated Employee	Site	School Year

Provision of School Nurse Services	School population
Subject	Grade Level

....

Agreement Reached On: _____9/29/72_____ _____Doris S. Bryan_____ _____
                                Date   Evaluator Signature   Evaluatee Signature

Who: All students and other personnel on school premises who present themselves to the
     Nursing office.

When: _____ continuous within school year. _____

Performance Criteria: Render first-aid and emergency care as required as outlined in

Administrative Bulletin 14 to those who present themselves for such service.

Measurement Technique: Numerical count on Nurses Daily report and reported annually

as required.

Methods, Strategies, Procedures and Techniques: Individual classrooms are supplied with first-aid

supplies (other school personnel provide first-aid in minor cases and refer those more

serious cases to the nurse's office). Notify parent or responsible adult if additional
medical or dental care is advisable.

Support Requirements: Facilities, equipment, first-aid supplies. Ancillary personnel

(nurse assistant and health aide.)

_____

Mitigating Factors: If Applicable: _____

_____

_____

....

To Be Completed at End of Evaluation Cycle
Degree of Achievement: _____

_____

_____

copies: 1 evaluatee
           1 evaluator

7-6-72

Fig. 8-1. Provision of school nurse services.

Evaluation Plan I

Objectives and Standards of Performance
for Student Progress and Professional Competence

Toda, Mary F.	Durant School	1972–73
Certificated Employee	Site	School Year
School Health Screening	K through 6th Grades	
Subject	Grade Level	

****

Agreement Reached On: ___9/29/72___ _Doris S. Bryan_ _____
       Date   Evaluator Signature   Evaluatee Signature

Who: Students in grades Kindergarten, 2 & 4 and students in grades 1, 3 & 5 who did not participate in the screening program in the school year 1971–72.

When: Completion dates in parenthesis following individual screening tests (see attachment)

Performance Criteria: 91% of eligible students will participate in screening program.

Measurement Technique: Numerical count of (total students who participated in the screening (total eligible program.

Methods, Strategies, Procedures and Techniques: Use of necessary appropriate equipment for each activity. Procedures – see attachment.

Support Requirements: Parental consent, personnel, specialized equipment. Principal's active support in providing authority for successful prosecution of program.

Mitigating Factors: If Applicable: Based on last year's experience, some parents will be difficult to contact or to obtain their full cooperation. This is sometimes common in low income communities.

****

To Be Completed at End of Evaluation Cycle
Degree of Achievement: _____

_____

copies: 1 evaluatee
            1 evaluator

7-6-72

Fig. 8-2. School health screening.

Evaluation Plan I

Objectives and Standards of Performance
for Student Progress and Professional Competence

Toda, Mary F.	Durant School	1972-73
Certificated Employee	Site	School Year

Referrals	K through 6th Grades
Subject	Grade Level

••

Agreement Reached On: _9/29/72_ _Don S Bryan_
                     Date   Evaluator Signature   Evaluatee Signature

Who: Students who participated in the SHANS screening program 1972-73 and other students who have suspected health problems.

When: Within three months after screening results are available to the nursing office.

Performance Criteria: Refer 91% of suspected health problems to an established private or community agency for assessment, diagnosis and/or treatment. To have 71% of students referred seen by a primary source of medical care.

Measurement Technique: Numerical count of students in need of care, of students referred, and of students who were seen by a provider of medical or dental care.

Methods, Strategies, Procedures and Techniques: Identify those findings that are one Standard Deviation beyond the norm (in those areas where normas have been established). Review individual student's health records. Arrange conference with parent (telephone, notes, home or nursing office visits). Conferences with parents and students, referrals for care, identity of available community resources, teacher conferences.

Support Requirements: Test results. Parents who will seek and obtain medical or dental care as necessary. Source of health care. Finances. Transportation. Time.

Mitigating Factors: If Applicable: Student and/or parent who do not appreciate the health problem involved. Possible insufficient family income. Lack of transportation. Based on last year's experience, some appointments for services were not kept.

*Primary source of medical care - that service which a child and to some extent his family receives when entering the community health care system and continues to receive in ambulatory or clinic type services.

To Be Completed at End of Evaluation Cycle

Degree of Achievement: _____

copies: 1 evaluatee
           1 evaluator

7-6-72

Fig. 8-3. Referrals.

Evaluation Plan I

Objectives and Standards of Performance
for Student Progress and Professional Competence

Toda, Mary F.	Durant School	1972-73
Certificated Employee	Site	School Year

Follow-up	K through 6th Grades
Subject	Grade Level

•••

Agreement Reached On: ___9/29/72___ _Chas J. Bryan)_ _____
                          Date   Evaluator Signature   Evaluatee Signature

Who: __Students who were referred for services.__

When: __Within current school year plus pick-ups in first semester of next school year.__

Performance Criteria: __71% of students referred because of suspected health problems will be__

seen by a provider of dental or medical services. Conference with teacher in 71% of

cases to inform her of findings.

Measurement Technique: __Numerical count of students referred for additional diagnosis or__

treatment. Numerical count of students who were seen by a provider for diagnosis and/or

treatment of the suspected health problem. Numerical count of teacher conferences.

Methods, Strategies, Procedures and Techniques: __Conferences with parents and/or students (notes,__

telephone calls, home and office visits). Conferences with providers of medical and

dental care. Conferences with teachers regarding possible classroom interventions that

might be beneficial because of physical findings.

Support Requirements: __Cooperation of parents, students, teachers and providers of medical and__

dental services. Finances. Transportation. Principal's active support in providing

authority for a successful prosecution of program.

Mitigating Factors: If Applicable: __Possible insufficient income of families and appreciation of__

parents to problem. Failure of the teacher to implement suggested interventions in

the classroom situation.

•••

To Be Completed at End of Evaluation Cycle
Degree of Achievement: _____

_____

_____

copies: 1 evaluatee
           1 evaluator

7-6-72

Fig. 8-4. Follow-up.

Evaluation Plan I

Objectives and Standards of Performance
for Student Progress and Professional Competence

Toda, Mary F.	Durant School	1972-73
Certificated Employee	Site	School Year

Health Education	K through 6th Grades	
Subject	Grade Level	

....

Agreement Reached On: _9/29/72_ _Doris J. Bryan_ _____
                         Date   Evaluator Signature   Evaluatee Signature

Who: Students, parents and teachers

When: Within school year.

Performance Criteria: Explain and interpret screening results to teachers and to parents for

91% of those students screened.   See attachment

Measurement Technique: List of subjects covered, numerical count of presentation time,

numerical count of those present and numerical count of teachers' requests for services.

Methods, Strategies, Procedures and Techniques: Various media such as films, slides, models, pamphlets

as available. Lectures, questions & answers sessions, resource persons will be

presented as appropriate. Books, periodicals, newspaper clippings, professional
journals will be available through the nurse's office.

Support Requirements: Time, availability of students and parents, teacher interest. Use

of principal's authority and support.

_____

Mitigating Factors: If Applicable: High transiency factor, release of personnel, teacher interest.

_____

....

To Be Completed at End of Evaluation Cycle
Degree of Achievement: _____

copies: 1 evaluatee
           1 evaluator

7-6-72

Fig. 8-5. Health education.

Evaluation Plan I

Objectives and Standards of Performance
for Student Progress and Professional Competence

Toda, Mary F.	Durant School	1972–73
Certificated Employee	Site	School Year

Policy Recommendations	K through 6th Grades
Subject	Grade Level

···

Agreement Reached On: _____9/_̲_9/7_̲_ _L̲o̲r̲a̲_ _S̲_ _B̲r̲y̲a̲n̲_ _____
                            Date   Evaluator Signature   Evaluatee Signature

Who: __Site administrator and SHANS Administration_____

When: __Continuous within school year._____

Performance Criteria: __Timely issuance of recommendations (where appropriate) to give____

sufficient advance warning to minimize or avoid health problems and illness crisis.____

Measurement Technique: __Numerical count_____
_____

Methods, Strategies, Procedures and Techniques: __SHANS staff meetings, Child Development Team____

conferences, random collection of suggestions, systematic study of Nurse's Daily____

Report to spot trends._____

Support Requirements: __Principal's support and interest. Teacher interest._____
_____
_____

Mitigating Factors: If Applicable: _____
_____
_____

···

To Be Completed at End of Evaluation Cycle
Degree of Achievement: _____
_____
_____

copies: 1 evaluatee
             1 evaluator

7-6-72

Fig. 8-6. Policy recommendations.

Evaluation Plan I

Objectives and Standards of Performance
for Student Progress and Professional Competence

Toda, Mary F.	Durant School	1972–73
Certificated Employee	Site	School Year

Process Control	K through 6th Grade
Subject	Grade Level

* *

Agreement Reached On: _9/29/72_   _David S. Bryan_ _____
                        Date   Evaluator Signature   Evaluatee Signature

Who: All students within the school during the school year.

When: Continuous during school year.

Performance Criteria: A health record for each student.

Measurement Technique: Smooth and timely allocation of resources to reach all previous objectives through the systematic use of records in the management and control of health problems.

Methods, Strategies, Procedures and Techniques: Record health information on individual Blue Health card. A "follow-up card" will be kept for those students with selected health problems. Data from health screening will be recorded as determined by SHANS administrator.

Support Requirements: Student records. Test results. Information from providers of medical and dental services.

Mitigating Factors: If Applicable: Lack of or untimely information from providers of services received on diagnosis and/or treatment of health problems.

* *

To Be Completed at End of Evaluation Cycle
Degree of Achievement: _____

copies: 1 evaluatee
           1 evaluator

7-6-72

Fig. 8-7. Process control.

objectives set for it, and the degree of achievement is based on the degree to which these goals have been met. Additional criteria for specific areas of evaluation are given as attachments to the plan.

Attachment to evaluation plan I

SCHOOL HEALTH SCREENING (Fig. 8-2)

Group screening of students in grades kindergarten, 2, and 4 and those students in grades 1, 3, and 5 who did not participate in the screening program in the school year 1971 to 1972.

1. School health check-up shall include the following:
   a. Stethoscopic examination (11-72)
   b. Phonocardioscan (10-72)
      Students: Third and fourth grade students and those fifth grade students that were not screened during the school year 1970 to 1971
      Conditions of performance: Testing on the PCS machine by a clinical technician
      Standards of behavior: Test passed (Those identified as failing are to be referred to the proper medical resource for further evaluation and treatment)
   c. Blood pressure and pulse (11-72)
   d. Anthropometry (heights and weights) within the first month of the school year and again during the last month of the school year
   e. Vision testing
      Conditions of performance: The modified clinical technique
      Standards of behavior: To be set by the testing agency
   f. Audiometry (12-72)
      Students: Those in the screening program and special referrals by teachers or parents of students in other grades
      Conditions of performance: Standard audiometric screening administered by certified, licensed audiometrists
      Standards of behavior: Normal hearing as indicated by passing the group, sweep or individual H-1 test
   g. Laboratory work (11-72): Hemoglobin, sickle cell test, blood typing
      Conditions of performance: To be contracted with a registered laboratory
   h. Urinalysis (11-72)
   i. Tuberculin Tine test (11-72)
   j. Health history (to be obtained at parent conference)
2. Screening activities done at each project school site

HEALTH EDUCATION (Fig. 8-5)

Performance criteria

1. Information pertaining to individual screening procedures will be explained by the nurse to 80 percent of the children who are participating in the SHANS screening program and other screening programs such as phonocardioscan.

2. In-service training or health issues and problems will be provided on a request basis.

3. Parent education—information on health issues will be scheduled as requested or as interest is shown.

4. Selected resource materials, pamphlets, books, and periodicals will be available to teachers upon request.

5. Assistance with curriculum planning and development on health subjects will be provided to teachers on a request basis.

Description of School Health and Nutrition Services (SHANS)

The aim of the SHANS Project is to demonstrate that coordinated utilization of school and community resources for health, mental health, and nutrition for children in selected Elementary and Secondary Education Act (ESEA) Title I schools will result in improved child and family health, better attendance, and improved communication and personal relations between the school, the home, and the community. This program was submitted and funded by Nutrition and Health Services of the Health, Education, and Welfare Department because parents, school personnel, and community health agencies have long been concerned with the many barriers in delivery and utilization of health services to schoolchildren, although many agencies and programs are available locally.

Each of four participating schools within the Oakland Unified School District has the full-time service of a school-community nurse, nurse technician, health assistant, and psychologist. The central office staff consists of the director, assistant director, dental coordinator, speech therapist, educational nutritionist, health educator, and half-time research consultant. Appropriate staff education programs are an important part of the program. Parent participation is encouraged and includes involvement in four school site councils and one central, overall body with close association to the Compensatory Education District Advisory Council.

Comprehensive medical, dental, psychological, speech, and nutritional screening with appropriately planned individual intervention is available for approximately 900 students each year of this three-year project. By the end of the third year of the project, all children in grades kindergarten through 6 will have been screened and engaged in treatment when necessary. Rescreening will be emphasized on second, fourth, and sixth graders in the last year of the project to compare with the child's earlier screening during the first year of the project. Data from the project will be available to assess health needs of children in deprived areas, the effectiveness of various follow-up strategies, additional roles for paraprofessionals and school nurses as school nurse practitioners, and the team approach. Innovations in health, dental, and nutritional education are being demonstrated and utilized for both elementary school pupils and their parents.

Second and fourth grade non–public schoolchildren who reside within the boundaries of these schools and meet the Title I criteria are also served. A breakfast program utilizing Federal Nutrition Act funds operates for approximately 1,200 children at the four schools. During the last year of the project, consultant services and some direct health education and health screening programs developed by SHANS will be available to schools outside the project. In addition screening will be offered to all younger siblings covered by Med-i-Cal in these schools.

9

ADMINISTRATION AND SUPERVISION IN SCHOOL NURSING

ADMINISTRATION PATTERNS

Administrative patterns for school health services vary, depending on the size of the school district, the services performed, and the personnel to perform these services. The board of education or the board of supervisors is the legally established representative for the agency. Their responsibilities include establishing general administrative policies and program policies, appointments of top administrators, and approval of budgets. The board of education advises the superintendent and is kept informed by him. They usually accept the recommendation of the superintendent and his staff on policies and programs.

Most boards of education are sounding boards for the community and have a specific time at each meeting for utilizing hearings on all types of issues. Boards usually meet on a weekly or bimonthly basis and, except for closed personnel hearings, are open to the public.

Boards of education members may be either elected officials or appointed by a city or a county board of supervisors. The chief executive in a school district is the superintendent of schools or in a health department, the director of public health. He usually is the official representative of the school district and administers the total school program. His decisions and activities are dependent upon assistant or deputy superintendents, directors, consultants, and supervisors of specific departments and principals of local schools.

Responsibility for the school health program is delegated to the superintendent of schools by the board of education. Overall responsibility for health services is assigned by the superintendent to an assistant superintendent, a director of special services, or coordinator of health. He in turn determines the specific responsibilities to the following members of the school health staff:

School nursing supervisor or school nursing director Initiates and administers the school nursing program within the framework of established policies and legal requirements for the school district. In districts where there are no nursing supervisors the duties are shared by the nurse, principal, teacher, and the administrative head of the health services.

School principal Administers the health program in the school within the framework of policies and procedures of the school district.

Classroom teacher Carries out her responsibilities for healthful living and health instruction for each child in her class according to the health needs of her individual class and the policies of the school.

171

School nurse Implements the nursing program within the school. School nurses are responsible to the school principals for their duties within the school and to the supervisor of nursing services or other designated authority for professional and technical activities.

School health programs in most cities and practically all rural communities, unless mandated by law, have restricted their periodic health examinations to referrals to the child's source of medical care rather than employing a school physician. This system, of course, is most desirable. Families then take their children not only for their usual physical examinations but also for other protective measures such as immunizations and correction of remedial health problems. Furthermore, when families get to know their doctor or clinic and the physician knows the children, the result is better service when the child becomes ill. A feeling of mutual trust does much for maintaining and improving the health of the schoolchild.

ADMINISTRATIVE AND SUPERVISORY PERSONNEL
The medical director

For many years it was believed that health or nursing services in any size school could not be provided without a medical director. This same belief was true in hospitals and many other institutions providing health services. The current position of the medical director in school health services has been appraised by Dr. Norman B. Schell* as follows:

> As general practitioners or pediatricians with active practices in their local communities, the part-time school M.D.'s (PSMD) are well equipped to handle many important tasks in school health and poorly equipped to cope with other important tasks. They are hired and publicized by the district as "part of the team" of health disciplines, viz., nurses, psychologists, physical and health educators, perceptual and speech therapists, etc., but their role usually entails many duties which they dislike and disapprove. These are usually responsibilities which are thrust upon them by local or state laws and regulations, e.g., "assembly-line" routine physical checkups in middle-income schools where the majority of students receive adequate primary medical care by private physicians in the community. . . .
>
> Since approximately 70 percent of school health services in the country are under control and direction of the State Education Departments (20 percent are under State Health Departments and 10 percent are under both departments), it is usually the pupil personnel office rather than the health office within the school that assumes responsibility for total health (physical and mental) care of the pupils, and the director of pupil personnel services generally delegates all procedures and operations (except physical examinations) in this realm to the other disciplines: nurses, psychologists, speech therapists, perceptual trainers, physical and health educators, etc. This director is commonly the captain of the team and the PSMD (part-time physician) is considered the player whose only wisdom lies in the use of the stethoscope, otoscope, and tongue blade.

Dr. Schell concludes his article with this paragraph.

> Review of recent trends in school health services reveals many areas which have become the domain of several specialized disciplines within the schools. Unless the current school physician acquires deeper interest and knowledge in these fields, his influence and value in the school will diminish. If he does not

---

*From Schell, Norman B.: School physician: a weakening breed, J. Sch. Health **43:**45, 1973.

improve his talents, he may be replaced by other personnel who are more available, more suited to the tasks, and more agreeable to the school budgets.

School medical directors or school physicians often come into the profession as a preretirement activity with no formal education or knowledge of what school health is all about. Often they are not willing or seem unable to realize the school physician is a specialist in his field and requires special study just as much as the internist, gynecologist, otologist, or other medical specialist.

Many physicians and educators are interested and study the problem of the physician in schools; hopefully they will recommend better means of working together and provide a more active commitment to school health services. Perhaps one approach, along with working as a team, would be for both the educator and the physician to study together more about learning disabilities and how to cope with this ever-increasing, difficult-to-recognize problem in school health. By bringing together the results of their research, the physician may be able to help the educator solve learning problems of pupils.

Using the hospital setting as an example, school health programs should be directed by a person with administrative experience and by a person trained to deal with groups of people, not on a one-to-one basis as are physicians. Most important of all, school nurses, *not* the physician, should supervise and teach nursing practices.

Medical and dental advisory boards

A growing trend in medical services that seems successful is the use of a medical or a dental advisory board comprised of specialists from the various medical areas involving children: the pediatrician, ophthalmologist, otologist, orthopedist, and psychiatrist. These specialists should be paid on a consultant basis for advice and assistance in their speciality. They should also thoroughly understand the purposes of the school health objectives. The scope of these boards' activities should truly be *advisory*; they may recommend policy and programs, but advisory boards do not set or implement policies and programs.

The school nurse administrator

Qualifications for the school nurse administrator, educator, and consultant are best expressed by the American Nurses' Association as follows*:

Legal

1. Holds a current license to practice professional nursing in the state in which employed.
2. Meets the state's certification requirements for the specific position.

Education and experience

In addition to those qualifications needed for staff positions:
1. Supervisory position
   a. Possesses a Master's Degree in School Nursing or Public Health Nursing from a college or university program accredited by the National League for Nursing, *or*

---

*From American Nurses' Association: Functions and qualifications for school nurses, New York, 1966, The Association.

b. Possesses a Master's Degree, earned by the completion of a curriculum appropriate to supervisory functions in a school health program. The following areas of study are recommended:
   (1) Principles and techniques of administration and supervision
   (2) School finance and law
   (3) Research procedures and statistical methods
   (4) Dynamics of human behavior
   (5) Community organization
   (6) School organization
   (7) Supervised experience in teaching and supervision.
c. A demonstrated successful experience in school nursing under qualified supervision.

2. Consultative position
   Same as for supervisory position, with addition of a successful supervisory and/or administrative experience. A special consultant should have had considerable experience in the specialty.

3. Educational position
   Same as for supervisory position, with the addition of:
   a. Preparation for teaching in schools of nursing
   b. Progressive experience in school nursing under qualified supervision, including staff, supervisory, and/or administrative experiences
   c. A degree not lower, and preferably higher, than the degree being granted by the program.

4. Administrative position:
   Same as for supervisory or consultative positions, with a considerable part of total experience in supervisory or consultative positions in school health service.

General and professional qualities and proficiencies

Same as for staff positions with the following additions:

1. A desire, with appropriate aggressiveness, to assume responsibility for upgrading school nursing practice and education for school nurses.
2. Willingness and ability to accept leadership as a professional nurse in the affairs of the school and the community.
3. The ability and the courage to assume leadership in determining the proper role of the school nurse and school nursing service within the school and community.
4. Creative ability and initiative in guiding the school nursing service.
5. Critical attitude directed toward positive and attainable health goals for children and youth.
6. Interest and ability to engage in research appropriate to school nursing, to evaluate research findings, and to make appropriate application of research findings for the improvement of school nursing practice and preparation of school nurses.

Human relations in school administration

Since World War II marked changes have been taking place in the theories and concepts of educational administration. There has been a growing emphasis on the personal aspects of school administration. According to Daniel Griffiths,[1] concepts of the functions and process of administration are quite different from what they were

---

[1]Griffiths, Daniel: Human relations in school administration, New York, 1956, Appleton-Century-Crofts.

ten years ago and will be much, much different fifty years from now, with stronger emphasis on working with people and better conceptualization of the tasks of education. School administration has long passed the day when it can be considered purely a technical skill of maintaining a plant, planning a budget, and assigning classes and classrooms.

The specialist in the school. To add to the complexity of the school administrator's job is the task of working with specialists who spend a few hours per week in the school to those who have full-time staff assignments. Specialists usually do not teach but bring special skills to aid the teacher in the job of working with children.

The specialist creates a difficult problem for the school administrator, who must evaluate a program in which he has little competence. The school administrator cannot be expected to be thoroughly competent in all specialized fields, yet he does have the responsibility for seeing that there are effective and smooth-running programs in his school. The limited time spent in the school by the specialist compounds the problem confronting the school administrator.

The school administrator. The understanding and support of the school administrator is the key to good school health programs. Yet, in these complex days of many pressures, the school administrator has little opportunity to explore in depth the current health and social problems facing children and youth or to determine the contributions that can be made by qualified school nurses to assist in solving these problems.

The school administrator is responsible for the execution of nursing policies, but the quality of performance of the school nurse in meeting her responsibilities is dependent on the nurse's own ability and professional preparation. To evaluate professional credentials places an additional burden upon the administrator; the school administrator must provide leadership and supervision in selection of nurses as well as determine sound philosophy and policies pertaining to school health.

School principal versus nurse. The universal problem brought up at every nurses' meeting from Maine to California is the "problem school administrator," and surely there are many. There are also many dedicated school principals vitally interested in the health of pupils. However, the problem principals usually are not committed to health services and are insistent that nurses sit in their offices at all times in case there should be a serious accident or illness at the school. The principal usually makes it clear to his total staff that he runs his school with "no questions asked."

The nurse in this situation will usually find these administrators feel and act similarly to the other specialists in the school. In cases like this, nurses must be aggressive and expressive. After many attempts at interpreting their role, they may find that they are able to do a few more activities that will be more of a service to parents and pupils. Written memos sometimes help. Compromise is also a good approach—"I tried your way, now how about trying mine?"—and document reasons and results.

It is most difficult to resist a persistent, sincere individual, particularly if the problems are being jointly worked out and involve the health of the schoolchild. Few school administrators can resist pressure from parents for programs that mean better service and better health for their children, and so enlist as many parents as possible in a variety of ways and let it be known that they have a voice in urging policy and program changes. Parent praise is always music to the ears of the nurse as well as the principal of your school. All these techniques should be practiced with professional and ethical behavior.

PRIORITY CONCEPTS AT THE ADMINISTRATIVE LEVEL

Much on priorities has been revealed in the current literature. Ruth Freeman and Edward Holmes, discussing priorities at the administrative level in public health, state*:

> Priorities at the directional or policy level are usually relatively broad. . . . At the administrative and operational level priorities are more specific: priorities may be allocated to cardiac patients with a first attack, or to follow-up care of school children in deteriorated districts of the city.
> The degree of priority assigned will depend upon:
> 1. Expected impact or potential.
>   A. Expected impact or potential of the service in relation to saving lives. . . .
>   B. The expected impact of the service in relation to improving health, preventing illness or disability. . . .
>   C. The expected impact of the program in relation to improvement of health practice and by implication raising the health level. . . .
> 2. The accepted obligations of the agency, as defined by law or incorporation statements. . . . The public health agency, by its nature, must be concerned with the health of all of the people in a community. It must consider the community as the patient. It cannot take concern for only one segment of the community, unless by so doing the maximum good for the total community is achieved. It must function within its defined obligations. . . .
> 3. Community readiness. In a country in which medical and related facilities are very scarce, preventive and health promotional services may be badly needed to raise the level of family health care. However, if the group providing service does not take into account the community's preoccupation with the need for curative services and give priority to these matters at a high enough level to assure the community of the helpful intent, there may never be a chance to go to the more sophisticated services. . . . By giving priority to programs for which the community is ready, it is possible to create a climate that will make it easier to move to the other programs later.
> 4. Public relations impact. Sometimes a program that is lower on the scale in some of the above categories may be moved toward the upper priority levels because it is a potential force in molding public opinion in relation to needed future services, or in reaching groups not now reached by services that belong to the whole community. . . . Certain school services may also produce this effect. If the health department is seen as property of all of the people, it is important to reach as many as possible with the services they need.

Henrik Blum and Alvin Leonard[2] discuss setting priorities in much the same way as stated by Ruth Freeman and Edward Holmes but add these items for consideration: (1) values and skills of employees, (2) values of those with vested interests,

*From Freeman, Ruth, and Holmes, Edward: Administration of public health service, Philadelphia, 1960, W. B. Saunders Co.

[2]Blum, Henrik L., and Leonard, Alvin R.: Public administration—a public health viewpoint, New York, 1963, The Macmillan Co.

particularly at the policy making levels, and (3) application of concepts to school nursing. Let us examine these concepts in the light of school services and specifically school nursing services.

Directional policy concepts

School health programs are generally described in school policy manuals with such general statements as "The objective of the health program is to provide the opportunity for every child to be in the best physical, social, and emotional condition to benefit from the educational process so that he may develop into a responsible, productive individual to meet the challenge of today's society." An addition to this statement might be "The school health program includes (1) school health services, (2) school health education, and (3) a healthful school environment."

Expected impact or potential. In school nursing the "expected impact or potential" means the optimum use of the nurse's time to do the greatest good in the nurse's particular school environment. In a school in a low socioeconomic ghetto the nurse might well need to spend much more time on first aid and health assessment of children to ensure the children's health in school. In another community the nurse might be spending more time in working with the school staff on developing a comprehensive educational counseling program on drug abuse.

Accepted obligations of the agency. The basic obligation of the school is education. All school nursing services must primarily assist children in their learning process. Services are directed toward promotion of health and prevention of disease. A well-clothed, well-fed child, who can see to read and hear the teacher, is more receptive to the educational process. Another component of schools' commitment to education is in health instruction. Children must be brought to know and respect the human body, human emotions, and the whole gamut of social relationships.

Community readiness. The needs of local communities are again reemphasized as an integral part of school health programs. Health services in schools complement the existing services in a community—they do not duplicate services. The involvement and endorsement of the school health programs by the parents, the medical community, and the department of public health is of vital importance for success.

Public relations impact. Often the dramatic school programs are given high priorities for public relations impact. The handicapped children program and the program for pregnant teen-agers, which affect fewer students, often receive higher priority than an immunization program that affects all students.

Values of skills of employees. Too often school nursing programs reflect concentration on areas of interest, skill, and experience of the nurse rather than the needs of the children in that school. To some degree this is true of all persons—the tendency to do what gives satisfaction results in the practices we do well. The nurse who is an excellent teacher will direct the school program toward health education. The research-minded nurse will probably spend much time on health records; the nurse with an epidemiological orientation will concentrate on a tuberculosis detection program, and so on.

Values of those with vested interests. School nursing is no better or worse than other disciplines in considering priorities dependent on "vested interests." Nurses may go into school nursing and stay on the job solely for personal reasons: "I want to go into school nursing so that I can be free to care for my children." "I want my summers off." "I've got tenure and this job pays well, so I'll stick it out until I can retire." "We do dental inspecting because we've got three dentists on our staff."

Comprehensive health screening

During the last few years comprehensive screening programs have been introduced in the schools. Several experimental programs have been funded by the Health and Nutrition Services of the U.S. Department of Health, Education, and Welfare. Twelve experimental programs have been selected throughout the country. Health screening includes medical, dental, speech, nutritional, and psychological components. Some of these programs are being done in neighborhood health centers, other programs by long-established clinics, and others within the school itself. These health screenings not only include the usual vision, hearing, and speech programs but also blood and urine testing, heart examinations, abdominal palpation, and posture and gait appraisal. These comprehensive screenings are by school nurse practitioners in many instances. An extensive health history and teacher observation are an important adjunct to these screenings. Parents are involved in these programs from their inception, and the results of follow-up on defects are excellent. A medical and dental advisory board is of great assistance in these programs. None of the projects is headed by a physician.

Data from the screening programs are available through computers for rapid and easy utilization by physicians, dentists, and other community workers. The teacher and other school personnel are provided with this same health data to assist them in directing the child's progress in school.

In a federally funded project at the University of Rochester a pupil personnel team of nurses, psychologists, physicians, teachers, speech therapists, etc., and a suburban elementary school worked together to explore ways the school district and pediatricians could cooperate. This was considered a successful project in meeting the major health needs of the schoolchild and was to be expanded to other elementary schools. Another problem, particularly in large cities, is that parents take their children to emergency wards of large hospitals or clinics for "on-the-spot" care of acute illness and do not return or follow through with a regular source of care because they do not have a family physician. Here again an alert school nurse practitioner can give valuable counsel and referral.

ADMINISTRATIVE RESPONSIBILITIES
Staff ratios

The determination of a staff ratio for an individual school is the responsibility of the school administrator. Discussions and articles about school nursing staffing ratios have always been vague and ratios have never really been defined. Staffing ratios as set forth in this book are also going to be vague and undefined.

For the past few years, school nursing ratios have ideally been set as one nurse to 1,200 pupils. Other authorities have stated one nurse to every 600 students. However, these ratios do not stand up in large city ghettos with a multiplicity of problems, in rural areas where some schools only have fifteen students and are 70 miles from the school nurses' headquarters, or in school districts where most pupils regularly see their pediatricians, dentists, and psychiatrists. The more widespread use of auxiliary nursing help and the expertise of the school nurse practitioner all add to the staffing dilemma. Then, too, the knowledge, skills, and experience of the nurse, the nursing program, and the commitment of the school administrator must be considered in determining the necessary number of school nurses.

New priorities for service must be set and school nurses themselves must take an active, intelligent role in determining the types and amount of activities feasible and meaningful for them to do in the time allotted to meet the health needs at their particular school.

Budgeting

The administrator or supervisor of school nursing services is often, and should be, involved in budgeting for services. Budget making should be based on needs, programs, and priorities for services. Usually a budget for nursing and health services is prepared and incorporated into the total budget for the school district or health department. It should be borne in mind that all monies are public funds and the superintendent or health official is responsible for expenditures.

Primary allocations include expenditures for personnel (both professional and clerical), travel, supplies, equipment and educational media, and estimates for new and innovative projects. There are usually experts in the school who can give assistance in preparing the budget, but it is important that the administrator of school nursing services understand as much as possible about preparation, financing, and final adoption and that the administrator keep a careful account of expenditures.

Cost accounting. A procedure utilized more and more by school districts is that of unit cost accounting. This means that the complete cost of each budget item is computed and compared with outcomes of service. Cost accounting, if used correctly, can be of benefit in setting priorities. For example, the cost of various kinds of parent contacts by nurses in relation to referrals completed may demonstrate that certain practices are outmoded and should be eliminated and methods more effective and less expensive to the district should be adopted.

Annual reports

One of the responsibilities of the school nurse administrator is to provide an annual report to the school administration and to the board of education. The reports can vary from a one-page summary of selective services to comprehensive printed reports covering total activities and programs.

One of the most consistently outstanding annual reports is published by the Denver Schools. It gives a complete account of services, programs, and philosophy of school health. An example of an annual report is given in the summary model at the end of this chapter.

Annual reports are most important in justifying services and in assisting parents and the public in understanding health needs and health programs within the schools. The school nurse administrator should plan for the annual report before the school year commences, and data-collecting forms should be thoroughly explained and written directions given to the staff as early as possible at the beginning of the school year. Forms should be simple and directly related to program and performance

Table 2. Frustrations of school nurses

Frustrations	Percentages
Lack of administrative understanding	47
Heavy case load	16
Clerical duties and simple first aid	16
Poor working conditions	8
Lack of prestige	8
Lack of parental understanding	2
No answer	2
Total	99

objectives. In some school districts a committee of nurses and administrators usually develop and review the data and make recommendations for direction and redirection of services for the next school year.

In this era of eliminating of services and cutting as many "extras" as possible, the annual report is an invaluable tool.

Job satisfaction

The satisfaction one derives from the work he does can be the most effective influence for good performance. If school nurse administrators apply the principles given in the section on implementing school nursing services, they are well on the way to ensuring satisfaction and maintaining high morale with the staff. However, an increasing problem is the diminishing of the school dollar and cuts in the nursing services.

School nurses receive satisfaction in (1) working with children and parents, (2) working with a variety of persons, both male and female, usually intelligent, and also dedicated to working with children, (3) freedom in planning one's own daily program within the school, and (4) promoting primary prevention of health problems by imparting health knowledge for a high degree of wellness. All of this means job satisfaction through working and helping others. Nurses usually are recognized and respected for the job they do in the school, which also adds to their satisfaction.

A necessary component in school nursing satisfaction is reassurance that school nurses need not worry about losing their livelihood. At present in many states, school nurses are in a teacher retirement program, not in social security, so that loss of a position also means loss of an adequate retirement income. The public, and some school administrators and teachers as well, rationalize that nurses "can always find a job." However, preparation for school nursing takes many years of specialized education, and the so-called available jobs usually provide less salary and less retirement security. This dilemma is definitely not a morale booster.

The school nurse administrator should encourage the staff (1) to be vocal in interpreting and defending their priorities, (2) to enlist the support of local, state, and federal agencies to provide specifically for nursing services in their appropriations to schools, (3) to inform parents of the suggested cuts or elimination of services and ask for their assistance and support, (4) to form an ad hoc committee to work together devising methods for action, (5) to work with school nursing and professional

Table 3. Satisfactions of school nurses

Satisfactions	Percentages
Service rendered	68
Personal relationships	16
Teaching	8
Seeing results	5
No answer	2
Total	99

educational organizations, and (6) to prepare a fact sheet pointing out the benefits to children of nursing services.

Nurse administrators should assist in all feasible ways. If possible, they should investigate and try to obtain outside or special funding for special nursing projects. They should provide opportunities for the total staff to assist with meeting these challenges and reassure their staff that their contribution to the health of schoolchildren is worthwhile and that these cuts in services in no way reflect upon the quality of their performance.

Nursing performance may diminish in such trying times; yet the administrator can be encouraging and optimistic but always keeping in focus the realities of the situation. At a recent health convention, nurses from Minnesota were wearing large green campaign buttons stating "Today's School Nurse Makes a Difference," and she does!

In a recent questionnaire given to 288 school nurses at a school nursing workshop that I directed, it was found that 47 percent stated their greatest frustration was lack of understanding by administrators and school staff and 68 percent stated their greatest satisfaction was from services; the next greatest satisfaction was from personal relationships (16 percent). There were two open-ended questions: "School nursing is most frustrating when . . . " and "In practice, the school nurse's greatest satisfaction is. . . . " The total results from the group are tabulated in Tables 2 and 3. Careful interpretations of these results give many clues to the work and philosophies of the nurse on the job.

IMPLEMENTING SCHOOL NURSING SERVICES

Quite often written programs and the reality of a given situation are far apart; this is one of the greatest problems for the nurse administrator. Principles for supervision include the following:

1. Selecting a competent staff
2. Clearly understood program objectives
3. Adequate and comprehensive orientation and continuing staff development programs
4. Worthwhile staff meetings with staff participation
5. Staff input—usually through committees on all aspects of the program: procedures, records of implementation of new programs—staff development, public relations, social
6. Supervision of nursing activities as a two-way learning experience

7. Written as well as verbal communications—clear, concise, and understandable —on all important programs and policies, that is, procedures book, special bulletins, staff agenda, and minutes of meetings
8. Be frank, honest, and deal fairly and squarely on all issues
9. Include the total staff, as well as the nursing administrator, in a sound public relations program
10. Staff evaluation and program planning—explained in detail in Chapter 8

Student nurse program

One of the obligations to the profession is to provide meaningful school nursing observations and experiences to students from nearby educational institutions. Student nurses spending a few hours or a few days in observation of various aspects of the school nursing program has little value and often leaves the student bored and preoccupied. If at all possible, student nurses should be assigned to the same school district for a specified number of hours. In California students must spend 180 hours of field experience in a public school before qualifying for a credential.

Detailed planning, meaningful experiences, and actual participation in the program are a must. In addition, students should only be assigned to nurses interested in the program and who are willing to exert the extra effort needed to work with students. Student nurse experiences must be educational and varied in nature, and students should not be accepted because the school district may believe it will receive extra school nursing services.

School nursing internship programs have been set up in several states in which the nurse works for a small salary while learning. These programs were successful and should be explored further; however, most have been eliminated because of cuts in all health services funds.

Student nurse field experience should be concurrent with academic courses or seminars with qualified instructors at institutions of higher learning. These instructors should personally visit their students to ascertain their needs and provide field supervision. Student nurse programs within the school should only be made available where there is an adequately prepared school nurse supervisor.

Certification for school nurses[3]

It has been said that school nurses should be certified or credentialed. The primary reason usually mentioned for this is that "teachers have to be certified," implying that because the nurse is in the school, she should do as a teacher does. This, of course, is impractical and unreasonable since a nurse is a nurse in school—she is not a teacher.

Certification of professionals at local and state levels is a priority to ensure continuity of preparation and appropriate preparation for quality service. For these reasons, certification for school teachers, school nurses, school administrators, school psychologists, school social workers, and school physicians has been successful in certain areas of the country. In other parts of the country certification practice is

---

[3]Woodruff, Margaret: Professional nurse viewpoint—certification of school nurses: three views, finis issue of School Health Review, September, 1969.

nonexistent or so riddled with politics and vested interests that it should be nonexistent.

In these changing times it would seem a better idea to have school nurses licensed by a national board. Setting up criteria for education and preparation for national examinations and licensing might be a next step. At present, certification requirements are so varied that any kind of national standard would be impossible. Some states have no requirements at all: other states require a range of from sixteen to thirty college credits and the diploma of nursing to five years of college preparation.

In New Jersey the new State Committee on Higher Education wishes to abolish all certification. Presently, thirty very specific credits are required for certification and must be obtained after three years of employment. If the nurse has the money, the fortitude, and three years of time, she may become certified. This does not guarantee a competent school nurse. By the time the nurse has acquired a permanent school nurse certificate, she has also obtained tenure.

In the state of Washington a move is afoot to provide certification on an individual basis. A conference is held with the nurse, the employing school administrator, and a representative of higher education. The nurse evaluates her academic preparation, her competencies, and identifies the areas that need emphasis. The employer expresses his preference, and the college representative outlines the courses needed to meet the requirements of the university. This program leads to a master's degree in school nursing and does give some flexibility.

LEGAL DECISIONS REGARDING SCHOOL NURSES

It is becoming more and more apparent that consideration must be given to some legal aspects of school health services and school nursing. Each state has its own educational code and health and safety codes that should be reviewed carefully by administration.

It is good advice that whenever there are doubts about the scope of nursing actions, legal consultation should be sought. Legal guidelines in the area of human rights and responsibilities are changing so fast that anyone who makes pronouncements on the subject is in danger of being outdated before he finishes his statement. Each state has a number of codes or state board of education rulings or state board of health rulings that will partially govern some of nursing actions. These will vary from a simple statement to many chapters in some of the more populous states. The California code says: "In all school districts there shall be instruction in health and physical fitness, including effects of alcohol, stimulants, tobacco, and narcotics on the human system. The State Board of Education shall cause to be prepared such study guides, materials, and reference lists as it may deem necessary to make effective the provisions of this section." Policies adopted by the local board of education have lawful effect and should be familiar to everyone working within the district.

Below are some of the cases which seem to point a direction for school health services.

The first concerns the authority of boards of education to employ nurses, dentists, and physicians. A number of cases have come into the courts involving the authority of boards of education to spend school funds for the services of nurses, dentists, and physicians. The courts are in accord in holding that, even in the absence of any specific statutory grant of authority, funds may be spent for such professional services provided that the duties performed are merely inspectoral and diagnostic. In the case of Hallett versus the Post Printing and Publishing Company, an injunction was sought to restrain the Board of Education of Denver from issuing warrants for the maintenance of the School Health Department in which it was employing physicians, dentists, and nurses. It was contended that the Board had exceeded its lawful authority because there was no statute authorizing the expenditure of public funds for such a purpose. The court refused to issue the injunction on the grounds that the Board was exercising powers necessarily implied. The court reasoned that the power of the Board to excluded pupils not meeting reasonable health requirements was undoubted; furthermore, the power to exclude such pupils implied authority to make requirements and to determine whether the requirements had been met. In both cases, expert advice was necessary. Moreover, the Board had the implied power to provide for the physical education of children. To provide such education, it was necessary to employ suitable persons to determine what was proper and beneficial for each pupil and to prescribe suitable exercises to overcome defects. The court was careful to point out, however, that the duties performed by the dentists and physicians employed by the Board shall not include medical or surgical treatment for disease. That would be to make infirmaries or hospitals of the schools. [*Hallett v. Post Printing & Publishing Company,* 68 Colo. 573, 192 Pac. 658, 12 A.L.R. 919.]

To the same effect is the decision in the case of the State versus Brown. The Board of Education in Minneapolis employed a nurse for one month to make an inspection of the physical condition of pupils in certain schools. The comptroller of the city refused to countersign the warrant for her salary on the grounds that the Board had no authority to employ her. The court held that the Board exercised an implied power. The court said, "The purpose of the school corporation is to maintain efficient, free, public schools within the city of Minneapolis, and unless expressly restricted, necessarily possess the power to employ such persons as are required to accomplish that purpose." Education of a child means much more than merely communicating to [him] the contents of textbooks. But even so, if the term were to be so limited, some discretion must be used by the teacher in determining the amount of study each child is capable of. The physical and mental powers of the individual are so interdependent that no system of education, although designed solely to develop mentality, would be complete which ignored bodily health. And this is particularly true of children whose immaturity renders their mental efforts largely dependent upon physical condition. It seems that the school authorities and teachers coming directly in contact with children should have an accurate knowledge of each child's physical condition for the benefit of the individual child, for the protection of the other children with reference to communicable diseases and conditions, and to permit an intelligent grading of pupils. These and other considerations convinced the court that the Board had the implied authority to employ the nurse for the purpose of inspection. [*State v. Brown,* 112 Minn. 370, 128 N.W. 294.]

Some schools do maintain clinics and they do it with specific legislative authority. In the absence of specific legislative authority, such practices have been challenged in the schools. The case involving the Board of Education of Seattle is an example. The court ruled as follows: "That the rendering of medical, surgical, and dental services to pupils is and always has been, we think, so foreign to the powers to be exercised by school districts or its officers that such power cannot be held to exist in the absence of express legislative language so providing." There is much in the argument of counsel for the school officers which may be considered as lending support to the view that such power ought to be possessed by the school district and its officers, but it is probable that counsel has many well-meaning people upon his side of the question. The legislature may give heed to such arguments, but the courts cannot do so. [*McGilva v. Seattle School District No. 1,* 113 Wash. 619, 194 Pac. 817, 12 A.L.R. 913.] In this particular case, legislative action followed which gave the school board the necessary authority.

As a general rule, boards of education under their general powers have authority to enforce regulations whereby pupils who are a menace to the health of their associates may be excluded from school. A North Dakota case ruled that, "Since attendance at the public schools is a privilege extended by the State, the State may, through properly constituted authorities, exclude from school all pupils whose presence in the schools would jeopardize the health of other pupils." Thus, pupils who are merely suspected of being affected with a contagious disease may be excluded from school. In the North Dakota case, for example, a survey made by the public health service of the federal government revealed that in a certain county there were 120 positive cases and 350 suspected cases of trachoma. The county board of health issued an order excluding the suspected cases from school. The court sustained the action of the health authorities and said, "The order of exclusion in the instant case cannot be said to be unreasonable. It only excludes those whose cases are positive and suspected, who are not at the time under treatment." The seriousness of the disease and its communicable character afford ample foundation for such an order. Even conceding that it may be doubted in the instant case whether the children in question are affected, the doubt is one that must be resolved in favor of the authorities charged with the serious responsibility of preventing the spread of the disease. [*Martin v. Craig,* 42 N.D. 213, 173 N.W. 787.]*

There seems little doubt that school nurses have good legal status within the public school system. The range of their activities will be governed by local and state regulations in addition to the code of ethics of their profession.

SUMMARY MODEL
Annual report of nursing services

The school nurse is a member of the educational team whose goal is to see that each child is in the best possible physical and emotional condition to benefit from his school experience and to reach his educational objectives. The school nurse works with parents and other community workers as necessary and often bridges the gap between the school and the home and between the school and various community organizations and health resources.

In some of the larger schools, or those with special health problems, the school nurse is provided with an assistant. The nurse assistant is trained and supervised by the school nurse. She performs minor first aid and initial vision screening, checks on immunizations and attendance problems, and transports ill or injured children, thereby releasing the school nurse to work more intensively with children and parents having special health needs.

Nursing staff

Total school nurse positions (includes supervisor, special programs and special projects)	47.8
Full-time nurses	44.0
Part-time nurses (4/5 time)	4.0

---

*From Ellis, Rulon: The school in society. In workshop proceedings for school nurses, Idaho State University, Department of Nursing, Pocatello, Idaho, 1970.

Part-time nurses (3/5 time)   1.0
All are assigned to eighty-eight schools or to special projects.

Total nurse assistant positions (includes special programs and special projects)   12.9
Full-time nurse assistants   2.0
Part-time nurse assistants   17.0
All are assigned to nineteen schools or special projects.

Health appraisals of all students. Nurses are responsible for promoting health examinations by the family's usual source of medical care and obtaining the reports or health inventories from the parent in order to detect those students who may have problems that need to be understood by the school staff. These reports help in the detection of those who may need guidance in obtaining adequate medical care. Teacher and parent observations are also an important source of this appraisal process. Screening surveys are done on all pupils in selected grades for common defects most efficiently detected in this manner; these surveys include vision, hearing, tuberculin testing, and, in specific schools, scalp ringworm, and heart defects.

Assistance to students with defects. Special assistance to handicapped children includes conferences with students, parents, the family physician, and other community agencies and recording and reporting of the problems for the benefit of others in the school program. The physical problems and prospects of correction are carefully determined for all students receiving special educational services. The school health services identify and follow-up all children eligible for care under Medi-Cal and Crippled Children Services.

Health supervision in school hours

The following health supervisory activities are included in this category:

1. First aid and advice for the sick and injured and supervision until the parents can be contacted and the child returned to the home
2. Supervision of safety practices on the school grounds
3. Inspections for communicable diseases and supervision of regulations for control of these diseases

Health instruction. The nursing personnel, because of their training and knowledge of the particular needs of the community, can be of great assistance to the teachers in health units. They also assist teachers in obtaining appropriate films, pamphlets, and laboratory and demonstration materials.

Community health responsibilities. The school is a part of a community enterprise. Therefore the nursing services exchange information and observations with appropriate persons or agencies and participate on many committees in order to develop and carry out cooperative health and welfare programs.

Research, reports, and evaluation studies. Specific programs within the nursing services are selected each year for evaluation and revision. Studies are done in areas of local or current interest and concern and the findings shared with other departments or agencies. New programs are initiated and evaluated.

Student programs. Each year about thirty-five student nurses are assigned to schools for field experience. Seven to ten nurses (health educators) and physicians in advanced public health programs obtain firsthand knowledge of school health services in the school district. Foreign visitors are sent to observe school health practices by federal agencies.

In-service education. Monthly professional education sessions are held for the nursing staff and guests. Participation in workshops and professional conferences is promoted. The nurses orient the teachers and parent groups to current aspects of public health at school meetings or conferences.

Selected services

ACTIVITY	DATA
First aid and care of emergency illness	
Nurses on call throughout the school day transport ill or injured children if no other means is available	Nurse or nurse assistant saw 269,827 individual students
Home visits	
Follow-up on health problems	17,673 visits by nurse or nurse assistant
Follow-up on ill or injured children regarding school oriented programs, that is, special education, attendance	
Vision screening	
Administered routinely three times during school—kindergarten, fifth, and eighth grades, all referrals by parents or teachers, all children new to district each year, plus special referrals	Performed 21,745 vision tests Follow-up on 2,852—failed eye test; 2,567 referred to eye specialist; 1,440 already under care (some referred for further care)
Hearing screening	
Done by school audiometrist	Follow up on:

Nurses do scheduling and follow-up and notification of parents	New detected losses—346
	Known detected losses—406
	   Referred to school otologist
	     New cases—132
	     Known cases—95
	   Referred directly for medical care
	     New cases—210
	     Known cases—144

Immunization	
School nurse, or nurse assistant, works with principal	Kindergarten or first grade Secured immunization data and follow-up on:
Polio and measles required by law	11,064 adequate immunizations 522 inadequate immunizations
Pupil heath records	
Individual health and immunization records are the responsibility of the school nurse—certain entries made by teachers and counselors	All children enrolled in the school district

Understanding individual health needs of the school. School district nurses are assigned to the same schools for a period of years so that they may personally become acquainted with pupils, parents, and school staff for more effective counseling.

Health education. The school nurse works closely with teachers in health education projects, programs, and correlates health services with classroom instruction.

Special health projects

Phonocardioscan project

Tested heart sounds of fourth and fifth graders—1,153 students	$2,300.00—funded by County Heart Association

M.C.T. project

Tested vision of 500 follow-through program pupils	$1,500—funded by Children's Vision Center

Health education slide project

Provided a series of colored slides with fact sheet for use in homes and classrooms, original script specifically for school district including a doctor's visit, a visit to the dentist, toothbrushing, rest and sleep, personal hygiene, selection of good foods, and vision and hearing screening	$400.00—funded by the County Cancer Society

Drug education project

For in-service drug education and a full-time drug coordinator	$49,000—funded by the state department of public health

ESEA summer dental project

Provided dental examinations and treatment for 500 children in ESEA schools Additional 800 through Medi-Cal	ESEA funded—$38,000 (approximately)

Dental health project

Provided dental health models and materials for non-ESEA schools	Funded by Dental Society Auxiliary—$800

These projects were written and implemented by nursing services staff.

Preparation of nurses

All nurses employed in this school district must have at least a baccalaureate degree, hold a public health nursing certificate, and have two years' experience in a local health department. These requirements are included in the special health and development credential required by the state department of education. Nurses are urged to have extra college courses in health education, counseling, guidance, and curriculum. They are required to attend planned orientation meetings on school nursing at least once a month during their first year of employement, and there are continuing staff education programs (once a month) on pertinent subjects related to school nursing. In addition, nurses are required to attend all regularly scheduled in-service education meetings for teachers.

10

PREPARATION FOR CHANGE

DIRECTIONS

In the preceding chapters transitional directions and redirections for school nursing have been discussed. New directions in programs, services, education, administration, and health instruction were based on sound research concepts. Changes in practice and innovative approaches were described.

School nursing, like any other profession, is in fact a profession only to the degree that its members are professional. Dorothy Tipple[1] in an address at a nursing conference borrowed this statement from the National Commission on Teacher Education and Professional Standards to suggest several premises for a professional:

A person who qualifies as a professional in any field:
1. Is a liberally educated person
2. Possesses a body of specialized skills and knowledges essential to the performance of his job
3. Makes rational judgments and acts accordingly; accepts responsibility for the consequences of his judgments and actions
4. Believes in his service to society
5. Assumes responsibility with his colleagues in developing and enforcing standards and abides by these standards in his own practice
6. Seeks new knowledge and skill in order to improve his practice

Please note that three of these six characteristics relate to education. Nursing education is moving quite rapidly and surely toward the achievement of professional preparation. Progress in school nursing is less clear. School nurses may be one of the best educated of any group within the nursing profession, but they also show the greatest diversity in educational preparation, which is significant. But perhaps even more significant is the fact that the diversity represents a wide range of nursing education. Some school nurses are graduates of associate degree and diploma programs with no additional preparation. At the other end, and the larger end, we have graduates of some of our finest baccalaureate and master's degree programs. In between we have registered professional nurses with conglomerate preparation in health and education. Some states have no certification requirements for school nurses. Others require a year of study beyond the baccalaureate degree.

Based on these facts, we can and should anticipate that the practice of school nursing will reflect the same range and diversity as the professional preparation

---

[1]Tipple, Dorothy C.: Overview of school nursing today—new dimensions in school nursing leadership, Washington, D. C., 1969, American Association for Health, Physical Education, and Recreation.

of the practitioners. As we move in the direction of improved academic preparation of school nurses and more intensive programs of continuing education, we can anticipate a higher level of professional practice.

At present there is an ever-growing body of knowledge to draw from. Barbara Baseheart[2] discussed the *musts, shoulds,* and *coulds* of school nursing. Let us hope all school nursing practice, regardless of professional preparation, has shifted through the musts and the shoulds to the coulds.

Musts Required by law (first aid, communicable disease control, screening).

Shoulds Interpretation of deviant behavior to teacher, parents, paraprofessionals (special talents, special wants).

Coulds Assist with classroom instruction, group work, family-centered programs, community projects, total school programs, and communication–health teaching.

PROFESSIONAL ORGANIZATIONS

Several professional organizations are interested in school nursing within the United States; these organizations are included in the following list:

1. American Nurses' Association
2. National League of Nursing
3. California School Nurse Association
4. American School Health Association
5. American Association for Health, Physical Education, and Recreation
6. National Council for School Nurses
7. American Public Health Association
8. National Education Association

What professional organizations do you belong to and why? What are the benefits to you? The cost of belonging to many is high—yet most nurses feel an obligation to the profession to join one or more.

1. The American Nurses' Association is the umbrella organization for all nurses, with sections for the various disciplines. Most significant for the school nurse is that belonging to this group provides a broad aspect for the entire profession. *The American Journal of Nursing* is their national publication. Two notable booklets published in 1966 specifically for school nurses and used extensively have been *A Rationale for School Nurse Certification* and *Functions and Qualifications for School Nurses.*

The American Nurses' Association is the nurses' official organization and should be the first that all nurses join and support. The state and local nurses' associations usually have school nurse and community nurse sections. These groups usually publish small journals and newsletters and are often bargaining agents for all nurses for higher wages, shorter hours, and more fringe benefits.

2. The National League for Nursing is primarily concerned with nursing education and has contributed much to school nursing through their accreditation program.

3. The California School Nurse Association is a group of highly dedicated, sincere school nurses who give time and untiring effort to further school nursing. They

---

[2]Baseheart, Barbara W.: Two-dimensional school nursing, Sch. Health Rev. **23:**23, 1968.

have recently organized the Department of School Nurses under the National Education Association. They are interested in nurses who are employed by boards of education. They have enlarged their services to many state organizations and provide consultation services, newsletters, and brochures describing their organization on school nursing.

4. The American School Health Association and its many affiliated state organizations was the first school health specialty group. It was originally confined to school physicians but now has more school nurses and health educators than physicians in its membership. It is a highly structured group working through study committees. This group is worth joining or having a school district join for its very fine *Journal of School Health,* edited for many years by Delbert Oberteuffer, Ph.D., of Ohio State University. This group emphasizes the concept of working as a team with all professional school health workers.

5. The American Association of Health, Physical Education, and Recreation has a very large membership, primarily from the physical education field. They have a very strong health education section and a newly organized Council for School Nurses. This group publishes a fine magazine, *School Health Review,* six times a year. In addition they have recently changed their name to the Association for the Advancement of Health Education and are anxious for more nurse members.

6. The National Council for School Nurses has a small, elite membership of nursing leaders from all over the country. All prominent school nurses have contributed their knowledge and skills to this group through writing, conferences, consultations, and studies. This group is particularly noted for their fine publications in school nursing: "New Dimensions in School Nursing Leadership," a report on school nurse leadership conferences; "Critical Issues in School Nursing;" and "This is School Nursing." They are presently preparing a report of a study funded by the United States Manpower Commission on curriculum for school nurses. They also present the Schering Award for the outstanding school staff nurse and the school nurse administrator each year.

7. The American Public Health Association has several sections of interest to school nurses—Maternal and Child Health, Public Health Nursing, and School Health. Besides excellent, well-organized national meetings, they publish the *American Journal of Public Health.* They have several regional and state subsidiary groups.

8. The National Education Association and its state and local groups is the top education association and many nurses in school are urged to join these groups, thus becoming more closely related to education. They also publish a journal and of late have been effective in legislative action for schools and negotiations for higher wages and more financing for public education.

All of these organizations and many others were usually formed because of a common interest and the need to exchange information for mutual growth. Most of these groups are middle-class, establishment-oriented, whose usefulness to the profession may not be as great as when they were organized. Because of the growing body of knowledge accessible to the professions, because educational institutions are providing more and more short courses and seminars for the professional, and because of the high costs of membership, many younger members of the professions are bypassing these organizations completely.

Selection of a professional organization

Any person contemplating membership in an organization should consider the following points*:

1. How much leadership is the organization taking in planning for comprehensive health care, including involvement of several professions, joint planning, and implementation?
2. What recommendations have been developed to implement health programs for disadvantaged children and youth?
3. How many members are concerned about health manpower shortages, and what special contributions and innovations are they encouraging for health programs of the future? How many think of the nonprofessional as only a threat to personal security?
4. Why are there few members from the minorities, yet at least 40 percent of the children in urban schools are from minority groups?
5. How many of the leaders of the organizations are under 40 years of age?
6. Are annual meetings providing the membership with the caliber and creativity of a vigorous, ongoing professional organization with emphasis on research?
7. Is enough leadership provided in promoting meaningful education and counseling programs in the critical areas of smoking, alcohol, misuse of drugs, family life, promiscuity, venereal disease, and student unrest?
8. Are school health priorities being set by vested interests rather than upon the needs of children?
9. Are they encouraging sound research in all areas of school health, are they adapting these findings or are they still following past outdated procedures?
10. What is being done by the organization to promote the school nurses' image as contributing members of the total school health team?

PREPARATION FOR CHANGE— PERSONAL PREROGATIVE AND PROBLEM

The following material is excerpted from a speech, "The Children's Charter and Mars: A Modern Dilemma."†

> We are constantly being made aware of these confusing and changing times. Some say that we really don't know what's happening to us, and that generates an uncomfortable feeling of disorientation.
> Even sociologists, who are used to explaining group behavior, complain that little can be counted on to endure from generation to generation.

Like our technological advances, our values and even the types of personalities we are supposed to admire are falling from their pedestals.

---

*Adapted from Bryan, Doris S.: Report of the president of the American School Health Association at the annual meeting, J. Sch. Health **40**:51, 1970.

†From Saylor, Louis F., Hodges, Fred B., and Vandre, Vincent E.: The children's charter and Mars: a modern dilemma, keynote address delivered at meeting of California School Health Association, Oakland, Calif., 1969.

The effects of the tragic assassinations of the Sixties will remain with us for many years, and the aftershocks will drastically alter the future of this country. Some of the issues posed by the new drug culture, by new styles of living, by new sexual mores, and by permissiveness in the arts are bound to have enormous impacts on the values, the traditions and eventually the history of American society.

The decade just ended has been one of protest over many issues. The Vietnam War leads the list. Poverty in the midst of affluence, taxes, and inflation follow close behind. Racism and the shameful slums of our cities, environmental pollution and lagging conservation—all are material ripe for protest. Add to these social problems the new life style of many youths, and the stage is set for drastic changes in traditional American values.

Our present time may be remembered as the beginning of rebellion by taxpayers everywhere. Tax overrides and school bond elections are being voted down with increasing frequency throughout the nation. The property tax, presently accounting for about 60 percent of the educational dollar in California, can no longer carry the traditional burden of being the keystone of educational finance.

Many other states are in much more difficulty than California. Teacher strikes, parent protests, and youth rebellions are becoming a common way of life for most urban schools. School health is part of this revolutionary scene. School nurses know firsthand the ferment, the excitement, and perhaps the fear of a changing professional world.

Knowing a problem exists and attempting to work out solutions is one approach to follow. Margaret Mead's comment that the greatest educational task is for us to educate our children for change becomes more relevant as the years go on.

All of us concerned with improvement in the quality of health must speak out aggressively. Health education of the most pervasive and enlightened nature must one day be recognized as a fundamental prerequisite to responsible citizenship.

As Dr. C. A. Hoffman, the president of the American Medical Association in his inaugural address stated:

> The next major advance in the health of this nation will come through health education, not through more doctors or more hospitals or new discoveries, but through public education in health care. We must persuade the American people that next to genetics, the single most important factor in health is life style, and that even more important than *environmental* pollution is *personal* pollution. . . . If we are heard, if our message is understood, it *will* improve the health of our people and it will free us from the burdens imposed by unreasonable expectations.*

We must have a substantial, productive health program to improve the quality of life of the human being whom we are supposed to be educating so he can live long, well, and understand himself. Whether this is done within the school, within the community, as a cooperative effort of both groups, or as an entirely new approach not yet even conceived is not the important issue. In any event, school nurses must play an important role.

The increasing emphasis upon health education, changes in the delivery of health services, a more vocal demand for adequate health care by the consumer are a

---

*From Hoffman, C. A.: The house of medicine, J.A.M.A. 221:483, 1972.

challenge to the total health team. This will demand the best that school nurses can give:

• Willingness to adapt to change when change is indicated
• Responsibility to their profession—nursing—and their specialty—school nursing
• Commitment to their own ideals and values
• Understanding and respect of the other's point of view
• Unselfish dedication

The health of children should know no national boundaries or political ideologies. In school nursing we have a common language that bridges the gaps in human understanding.

SELECTED READINGS

American Nurses' Association: Functions and qualifications for school nurses, 1961, ANA School Nurses Branch, Public Health Nurses' Section.

American Nurses' Association: School nursing practice, a guide for evaluating, implementing and improving the functions of school nurses, 1961, New York, ANA School Nurses' Branch, Public Health Nurses' Section.

American Red Cross: First aid textbook—multi-media approach, 1970.

American School Health Association: Mental health in the classroom, J. Sch. Health September, 1963.

Basco, D.: Evaluation of school nursing activities, Nurs. Res. 12:212, 1963.

Beacham, R., and Hesle, M.: A color-blind testing program in the Baltimore City Public Schools, J. Sch. Health 35:460, 1965.

Benell, F.: The role of the school in venereal disease control, J. Sch. Health 25:258, 1965.

Blum, H.: Vision screening for elementary schools—the Orinda story, Berkeley, 1959, University of California Press.

Bryan, Doris S.: Project Head Start—implications for school nurses, Calif. Sch. Health 2: 26, 1966.

Bryan, Doris, and Cook, Thelma: Redirection of school nursing services in culturally deprived neighborhoods, Am. J. Public Health 57:1164, 1967.

California State Department of Education: A guide for vision screening of school children, rev. Sacramento, 1972.

California State Department of Education: Drug abuse: a source book and guide for teachers, Sacramento, 1967.

California State Department of Public Health: Hearing testing of school children and guide for hearing conservation programs, rev., Sacramento, 1972.

Cauffman, Joy G., Petersen, E. L., and Emrick, J. A.: Medical care of school children, Am. J. Public Health 57: 1967.

Christy, T. E.: Portrait of a leader, Nurs. Outlook 18:50, 1970.

Coles, Robert: Children of crises, Boston, 1967, Little, Brown & Co.

Cromwell, G. E.: School nursing, Philadelphia, 1963, W. B. Saunders Co.

Cruickshank, W. M., and Orville, J. G.: Education of exceptional children and youth, ed. 2, Englewood Cliffs, N. J., 1967, Prentice-Hall, Inc.

Curtis, A. C.: National survey of venereal disease treatment, J.A.M.A. 186:46, 1963.

Davis, James A.: Education for positive mental health, Chicago, 1965, Aldine Publishing Co.

Doster, M., McNiff, A. L., Lampe, J. M., and Corliss, L. M.: A survey of menstrual functions among 1,668 secondary school girls and 720 women employees in Denver public schools, Am. J. Public Health 51:1841, 1961.

Dunphy, B. A.: In defense of school nurse's aides, Am. J. Nurs. 66:1338, 1966.

Editorial: School health education: A public health concern, Am. J. Public Health 57: 2061, 1967.

Florentine, H.: The preparation and role of nurses in school health programs, New York, 1962, National League for Nursing.

Fredlund, Delphie J.: The route to effective school nursing, Nurs. Outlook 15:24, 1967.

Freeman, R.: Public health nursing practice, ed. 3, Philadelphia, 1963, W. B. Saunders Co.

Gabrielson, Ira W., Levin, L. S., and Ellison, M. D.: Factors affecting school health follow-up, Am. J. Public Health 57:48, 1967.

Gallagher, J. Roswell: Medical care of the adolescent, New York, 1966, Appleton-Century-Crofts.

Growth patterns and sex education, J. Sch. Health May 1967.

Guthrie, Helen A.: Introductory nutrition, ed. 2, St. Louis, 1971, The C. V. Mosby Co.

Hanlon, J. J., and McHose, E.: Design for health; the teacher, the school and the community, Philadelphia, 1963, Lea & Febiger.

Havighurst, R. J.: The learning process, Am. J. Public Health 51:1694, 1961.

Hodgson, W. R.: Audiometric screening and threshold norms, J. Sch. Health 38:373, 1968.

Jacobson, Edmund: You must relax, New York, 1963, McGraw-Hill Book Co., Inc.

Louria, Donald B.: The drug scene, New York, 1968, McGraw-Hill Book Co., Inc.

Obertenffer, D.: Health and education—an appraisal, J. Sch. Health 34:184, 1964.

Radke, M. L.: What does the teacher expect of the school nurse? Nurs. Outlook 13:33, 1965.

Randall, Harriet B., Cauffman, J. G., and Shultz, C. S.: Effectiveness of health office clerks in facilitating health care for elementary school children, Am. J. Public Health 58:897, 1968.

Redl, F.: When we deal with children, New York, 1966, The Free Press.

Ritchie, Jeanne: School nursing: a generalized or a specialized service, Am. J. Public Health, 63:1251, 1961.

Roberts, Doris, et al.: Epidemiological analysis in school.populations as a basis for change in school nursing practice, Am. J. Public Health 59:2157, 1969.

Russell, R. D., and Robbins, P. R.: Health education and the use of fear: a new look, J. Sch. Health 34:263, 1964.

Savitz, R., Valadin, I., and Reed, R. B.: Vision screening of preschool children at home, Am. J. Public Health 55:1555, 1965.

Simon, Helen: A look at secondary school health, Nurs. Outlook 16:42, 1968.

Sliepcevich, Elena: Health education. A conceptual approach to curriculum design, St. Paul, Minn., 1967, 3M Education Press.

Tipple, Dorothy: The school nurse as a counselor, Am. J. Nursing 63:110, 1963.

Trice, Harrison: Alcoholism in America, New York, 1966, McGraw-Hill Book Co., Inc.

U. S. Public Health Service: The health consequences of smoking, Washington, D. C., 1972, U. S. Department of Health, Education, and Welfare.

Wagner, Marsden G., Shultz, C. S., and Heller, M. H.: A study of school physician behavior, Am. J. Public Health, 58:517, 1968.

Wayne, Dora: School nursing and team teaching, Nurs. Outlook 17:7, 1969.

Wheelis, Allen: The quest for identity, New York, 1958, W. W. Norton & Co., Inc.

Wilson, Charles C., editor: School Health Services, ed. 2, Washington, D. C., 1968, National Education Association and the American Medical Association.

INDEX